ADVANCES IN WORKING WITH WEIGHT

IS THERE A FUTURE FOR BARIATRIC SURGERY?

TOM TAYLOR

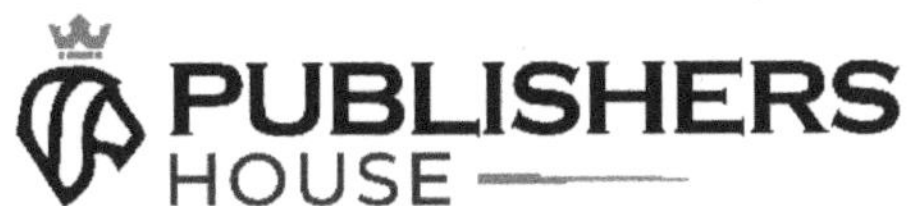

Hotline: +44 20 4614 9582

Email: sales@publishershouse.co.uk

Ordering Information:

Quantity sales. Special discounts are available on quantity purchases by corporations, associations, and others. For details, contact the publisher at the address above.

Printed in the United Kingdom.

DEDICATION

To Joy, Anna and Beth.

CONTENTS

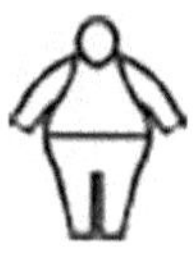

INTRODUCTION

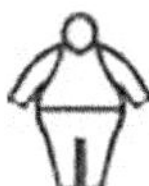

A century ago, the 12 major causes of death were influenza, tuberculosis, smallpox, poliomyelitis, staphylococcus, streptococcus, cholera, measles, plague, pertussis, leprosy, and malnutrition, out of which the major underlying cause was an infection.

Today, the majority of mortalities are due to high blood pressure, high blood cholesterol, and diabetes mellitus. This eventually leads to the major twelve killers: coronary artery disease, heart failure, arteriosclerosis, stroke, peripheral vascular disease, diabetes complications, dementia, cancer, liver disease, COVID-19, influenza, and lung cancer. In all of these ailments—with the exception of lung cancer—a major contributing factor is obesity.

The diseases of the first half of the 20th century were largely overcome by vaccination and antibiotics. There is a potential resolution to the current major killers. But this has not yet been grasped, and the prevalence of all of them is rapidly increasing, as obesity has now become the major underlying problem.

Obesity is a complex disease, a significant public health problem involving the accumulation of an excess of body fat, which ultimately impairs all of the above-listed major health disorders of the present day. There are multiple factors involved, such as hereditary, psychological, behavioral, and family factors, and a lack of physical exercise. However, unhealthy eating remains the major factor.

Obesity, in a literal sense, refers to an excess of body fat. An excess of body fat is defined as a total body mass index (BMI) in excess of 25 kg/m2 or a body weight of 20% or more above the ideal body weight. Some 50 million adults in the United States are obese by this definition.

Of these, eight million have a body mass index of over 40 kg/m2. This means that they suffer from severe or morbid obesity, the risks of which are life-threatening. This number has doubled in the last 10 years and is increasing rapidly. Although body mass index (BMI) is most commonly used to diagnose obesity, modern thought alludes to the quantity of fat in the body as being the most accurate parameter. These two mathematical parameters are commonly related in their outcomes. For most people, the body mass index provides a reasonable and workable index of the degree of obesity.

Weightlifters and extremely muscular individuals may have a high BMI. But they are carrying most of their weight as muscle and not as body fat. Waist circumference is also used as an indicative parameter of obesity. Males are particularly prone to gain weight around their waist, and weight-related problems do correlate with waist measurements of over 40 inches.

Basically, the physics of the situation comes down to the laws of thermodynamics. The laws of thermodynamics indicate that the more calories you eat and do not burn off, the more weight you will gain. In other words, "energy cannot be created or destroyed but only transformed from one source to another." This implies that extra ingested calories are converted into body fat.

Calories not burned off by hard physical labor or exercise are stored in the body as fat. Fewer physical jobs have made a huge impact on body weight. Two hundred years ago, canals were physically dug by shoveling soil. Road construction, building, and farming were done by hand.

Now, digging is done by powerful tractors. The workplace for many has also become sedentary, sitting in front of a computer all day. We don't walk because the use of the car has become ubiquitous. We use elevators and escalators, drive to restaurants, and mostly rely on domestic delivery vehicles to deliver precooked foods and other products.

Unhealthy diet is the main cause of the obesity crisis and is something we can all do something about. A diet high in sugar and fat, as in fast food diets, is the most dangerous contributory factor, and sugar is the main enemy. These foods are invariably accompanied by sugar-laced drinks. Restaurants provide oversized portions, often lacking in fruits and vegetables.

Eating solids is more protective than drinking large volumes of high-calorie soda. A can of Coke contains nine teaspoons of sugar. Alcohol is also calorie-laden at 8 calories per gram. So, drinking pints of beer at 250 cal or more each soon packs on the calories and increases abdominal fat and waistline dimensions.

Rarely does obesity have an underlying medical cause; the vast majority of cases are purely and simply due to eating more calories than you burn up. There are diseases that cause it: an underactive thyroid, Cushing's syndrome, and the rare Prader-Willi syndrome, which produces gross obesity.

Lack of mobility produced by osteoarthritis of the knees and hips prevents normal activities and predisposes to weight gain. Certain medications produce weight gain: steroids, particularly female hormones; some antidepressants and anticonvulsants; diabetic medications; and some beta blockers. Exercise and walking are discussed later at length. They are essential attributes, but don't burn up massive numbers of calories. And they are not, in themselves, the solution.

They also rely on access to parks, gymnasiums, sports facilities, country walks, and exercise clubs, which are frequently not available to many in the population. Too many people are now so focused on surviving economically in a "fast forward" world that time for exercise has long since been lost.

The United States is a very body-conscious country. Its public face, as depicted on magazine covers, in movies, and on television, is of youth, vitality, and sexual attractiveness. In reality, however, fewer and fewer Americans are now resembling this hallmark.

Body Mass Index	**Weight in Kilograms/ (Height in Meters) Squared**
Overweight	BMI > 25
Obese	BMI: 30–40
Morbidly Obese	BMI > 40

CHAPTER 1: THE NATURE OF THE PROBLEM

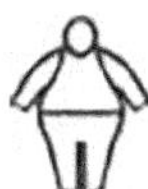

Obesity is more than a cosmetic problem: it is, as stated, the direct cause of a host of medical problems that are the biggest killers of American citizens today. The three most important problems associated with obesity are high blood pressure, high blood cholesterol, and diabetes mellitus.

This trio is often referred to as "syndrome X." Many millions of Americans suffer from syndrome X, the components of which are all linked to sugar intolerance and insulin resistance. This collection of problems now represents the number one public health initiative facing Western society. The disorder is much more common than cancer and COVID-19. Unfortunately, it is the mechanism by which we, in Western society, have created a new constellation of killer diseases. Due to this, we all suffer to a variable degree, which aggregates from a young age.

SYNDROME "X"

- Hypertension
- High blood cholesterol
- Diabetes mellitus

Consequences of Syndrome "X"

- Coronary artery disease
- Stroke

- Complications of diabetes
- Cancer: breast, colon, and ovary

LIFESTYLE

As stated previously, current lifestyle and behavior are largely responsible for this problem. The lifestyle is sedentary, and over the past century, technological developments have almost completely removed physical exercise from our day-to-day lives. In association with diet, this lifestyle sets the scene for the foremost killers of the day, which herald these 12 dominant diseases. The syndrome now affects not only the elderly or the middle-aged but also has a huge effect on children and teenagers.

CHANGES IN THE PAST CENTURY

Humankind has evolved over millions of years. But only in the last century have changes developed at an unrelenting pace, never before experienced. We have walked the roads to and from our destinations, day in and day out, for hundreds of thousands of years. In the past few thousand years, the fastest mode of transportation has been the horse. In the past century, we have developed the technology to travel the world in a day: from New York to Australia.

We have also become dependent upon mechanization in every walk of life: buses to school, cars to work, engines to dig the soil, to build roads and buildings, and manufactured goods. The effect of lying in front of a screen, eating and drinking carbohydrate-laced foods, has been to create a completely new model of humanity.

Our supermarket shelves are packed with cheap, mass-produced, good-tasting, readily available food, which is very high in calories. These foods are constantly attractively displayed in advertisements on the televisions to which we have become glued. And they are stacked with extra sugars to improve their taste.

GEOGRAPHY AND WESTERN LIFESTYLE

Interestingly, people who migrate to the United States from poor areas such as Latin America and Asia adopt Western lifestyles and become obese. And thus develop, over time, the diseases that now afflict Indigenous Americans.

Improved nutrition has done much to enhance human performance, physical and possibly intellectual. But modern nutrition has also created syndrome X, which is now killing us by underpinning the vast majority of today's fatal illnesses.

Think of a 1-pound bag of refined sugar; think of 150 bags of sugar in a pile. This is how much sugar the average person now consumes per year compared with a century ago. Cans of soda contain about 200 calories per drink, all of which are packed with sugar-refined carbohydrates. There is the equivalent of nine teaspoons of sugar in a can of soda.

SUGAR IS THE MAJOR CAUSE OF THE PROBLEM

Eating our way through this mountain of sugar is the primary cause of heart attacks, vascular disease, strokes, and diabetes. Other health problems that ensue are breast and colon cancer, menstrual abnormalities (polycystic ovary syndrome, which is also associated with female infertility), unwanted body hair, and acne.

Inflammation of the liver, increased tendency for blood to clot and produce thrombosis, and depression of the immune system may also result. These disorders are those of the 20th century, those of modern living, and those that can be dealt with. Coronary artery disease, stroke, and diabetes were all rare in the 19th century. Admittedly, many people died at a younger age, often of infectious diseases such as tuberculosis and pneumonia. There has been a complete transition in the categorization of the pattern of fatal disease.

THE WESTERN DIET

The common gastrointestinal conditions that surgeons treat today are all self-induced by the high sugar, low fiber diet. Gallstones, diverticular disease, appendicitis, hemorrhoids, and lung cancer are extremely rare in Central Africa—a region where a diet high in fiber and unrefined carbohydrates is prevalent. Take the Central African citizen out of his own environment and put them into the United States, however, and he will soon develop the same disorders as those that afflict the American population.

GASTROINTESTINAL DISEASES CAUSED BY SUGAR

- Gallstones
- Diverticular disease
- Appendicitis
- Hemorrhoids
- Colon cancer

Taking hunting from the "Hunter-Gatherer" equation, our earliest ancestors probably ate foods similar to those eaten by apes and monkeys. These were berries, fruits, shoots, nuts, tubers, and other vegetation in the forests of Africa. Most of these plants were relatively low in calories and took constant work to collect them, and also to stay alive.

Early humankind began eating meat some 2½ million years ago. And the environmental record shows that the human brain became remarkably bigger and more complex at about the same time. The incorporation of animal matter into the diet played an essential role in human evolution and development. The fatty acids found in meat also play an important role in brain growth and development.

The high concentration of nutrients in meat also gave humans some rest from consistently gathering and eating vegetation. In parallel, the growth of the brain produced guile, cunning, and organization. This led to the development of technology, socialization, and community living. The meat that our ancestors ate was high in protein and low in fat, less than 4%. Also, the supply was sporadic, and a lot of energy was expended in catching it, leading to a lean body habitus.

CHAPTER 2: THE BASIS OF OBESITY

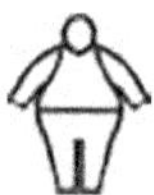

LAWS OF ENERGY

Sir Isaac Newton, the father of modern physics, stated that energy cannot be created or destroyed but only converted from one form to another. The law of conservation of energy states that the total energy in an isolated system remains constant over time.

Energy exists in many different forms: oil and food are forms of chemical energy. Burning oil permits planes to fly, cars to run, houses to be heated and cooled, and electricity to be generated. Burning food permits us to live, run, walk, talk, and do our many lifetime activities. The energy that isn't actively being burned in a plane or a car is stored in the fuel tank. Oil is a form of fat: when the tanks are empty, the vehicle stops.

SOURCES OF ENERGY

Mankind derives energy from three sources: protein, carbohydrate, and fat. We are extremely efficient in the collection, storage, and utilization of energy, much more so than planes or cars. The energy taken in food is either utilized or stored.

In the process of staying alive, maintaining our bodies and our body temperatures, we use energy of the order of 1500 calories per day. When we work, play sports, and partake in other activities, we burn up additional energy needed for these physical processes. We can easily utilize 2000 to 3000 calories per day (differences in calorie needs exist for men versus women).

In addition to the above, physical exercise, for example, riding a bicycle for an hour, typically burns only 300 to 400 cal. However, exercise is important in the energy equation and in the weight loss equation, though, in itself, it is not a potent source of weight reduction.

According to Newton's laws, any energy that our body does not burn, it stores. Protein provides 4 calories per gram, carbohydrates likewise, whereas a gram of fat contains 9 calories. The human body has fuel tanks like a plane or a car. But unlike the latter, these fuel tanks of the human body are made entirely of stored fat. And the overall ability of the body to store them is absolutely huge.

BASAL METABOLIC RATE

- Females: 1,200–1,500 calories.
- Males: 1,500–2,000 calories.

ENERGY STORAGE

The body does not function as a storage organ for protein. Weightlifters and muscle men store some energy, and they increase muscle mass, but not a lot. Likewise, the body is a poor storage organ for carbohydrates. There is some carbohydrate in muscle, and about 150 g is stored in the liver as a chemical called "glycogen." The body stores glycogen at about 600 calories, or the equivalent of about two hours of riding on the bike. Clearly, after two hours on a bike, we do not collapse into a state of energy depletion; we begin instead to use fat. The fat stores of the body are not only extremely efficient; they have the potential to be huge.

If we eat more calories than we burn—Newton's laws again—we store the excess energy, not as protein or carbohydrate but as fat. Unlike the fuel tanks on the vehicle, unfortunately, the fat stores in men do not replenish once they have had a large meal or taken in energy for a long journey; they can just keep on growing and can become enormous.

FAT IS THE VEHICLE OF ENERGY STORAGE

A morbidly obese subject does not have a basic frame size much bigger than that of a skinny person. He or she has the same amount of bone, a little more muscle, the same size brain, the same lungs and guts, and a little bigger heart for all the extra work it has to do. If the basic frame of a 600-pound man is 150 pounds, then he is carrying 450 pounds of fat and carrying it 24 hours a day—every time he moves, every time he walks, every time he climbs stairs. That is the equivalent of carrying about four large sacks of grain on his back every time he moves. These "sacks of grain" strain the heart, the muscles, the bones, and the joints. And they provide the basis for the vast majority of today's killer diseases.

Excess calories are rapidly converted to fat because calories cannot be lost if they are not burned. As fat contains 9 calories per gram, a steady excess caloric intake over our need of 1000 calories per day will lead to a weight gain of approximately 100 g per day or about two pounds per week.

Not much? Well, two pounds per week is one hundred pounds a year. An excess of 1000 cal per day is easily achieved and amounts to only four cans of soda or four small chocolate bars. And remember, it takes over two hours of cycling to burn off. Thus, consistently eating just a little in excess of one's needs can have profound consequences, particularly in the long term.

CARBOHYDRATES PRODUCE BODY FAT

In the process of food absorption and metabolism, excess carbohydrate intake is converted into fat and stored as such. Similarly, alcohol, which is energy-dense, with 8 calories per gram, is also stored as fat; even protein excesses may be stored as fat.

THE OBESITY INDUSTRY

In general, therefore, it is true to say that individuals who eat in excess of their needs will tend to be overweight, and those who do not eat enough will tend to be underweight. Seventy percent of Americans are overweight, and very few are underweight.

In consequence, weight control and obesity management are among the largest industries in North America. It is estimated that about one-quarter of the population spends about $50 billion on weight control each year.

Approximately 20% of the population describe themselves as being on a form of diet, and three-quarters of teenage girls try to control their weight or to lose weight. The vast majority of obese children become obese teenagers. Most obese teenagers become obese adults and remain obese throughout their lives.

Once the thermostat of weight creeps up to an elevated level, it rarely stabilizes back to normal in the long term unless some major intervention takes place permanently to affect the equation. And that, currently, means major medical or surgical intervention to reduce food intake and alter the underlying metabolic process.

SUGAR IS THE ENEMY

Historically, much emphasis was placed on the low-fat diet. The philosophy was often one of avoiding fat and giving "carte blanche" to the ingestion of carbohydrates. This has now been completely turned around, initially by the pioneering work of the late Robert Atkins, who popularized the low or "no" carbohydrate diet. When his work was introduced, his philosophy flew in the face of established thinking and was soundly condemned in many academic circles. But the proof of the pudding, in particular, was in the eating!

The bottom line for millions has been that the Atkins diet results in weight loss and even a reduction in cholesterol and amelioration of obesity and syndrome X. Sugar is the enemy; sugar is toxic, but recent studies have shown that the Atkins diet is far from the ideal solution, as this will be discussed below.

SUGAR AND INSULIN

Sugar is an easily absorbed and pleasant-to-eat source of rapid energy, but it has adverse effects by directly stimulating insulin production. Insulin has a direct causal effect on our bodies' ability to store excess sugar as fat, and it inhibits the mobilization of previously stored fat. In addition, insulin signals our livers to make cholesterol. That is why even when eating the high cholesterol content foods of the Atkins diet, levels of blood cholesterol may fall since there is less insulin production.

Diabetic patients have significantly higher total cholesterol and triglyceride levels than the normal population. It is for these reasons that modern diets like the Atkins diet, the South Beach Diet, and the Sugar Busters diet drastically reduce the amount of refined carbohydrates that can be consumed.

COUNTING CARBS

Counting carbs has become a powerful fixture in the economy and in society at large. Some 586 distinct new carbohydrate foods and beverages hit the grocery shelves in the first decade of the millennium, bringing the total over recent years to 1558 new entries. It is having a significant effect on the food giants as "carb watching" would appear to be here for the long term.

Things need to change! It is possible that the effects of carbo-counting are beginning to be established in America. It has been reported in recent years that, after many years of weight gain, the number of overweight adult Americans fell one percentage point to 59%. However, this is a minor incursion.

In parallel, in fast food restaurants, the total number of orders rose 12%. All the while, French fries consumption fell 10%. National potato production has also recently fallen by 5%. Present-day food containers, drinks, and restaurant meals all display detailed nutritional contents of their products, from fat, carbohydrate, and protein down to vitamins and minerals. And this is a move in a positive direction.

CHAPTER 3: THE CONSEQUENCES OF OBESITY

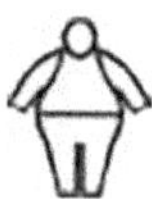

DIABETES IN CHILDREN

The presence of obesity stimulates the development of Type 2 diabetes, previously regarded as the adult form. Even in children and adolescents, diabetes is increasingly being observed. In affected children and adolescents, the type of diabetes is changing rapidly. In the past, it used to be that children got more aggressive and often inherited Type 1 diabetes.

Now, in addition, they are rapidly developing Type 2 diabetes. In a 10-year period, there has been a staggering 500% increase in Type 2 diabetes in children. And these children are invariably obese. The prevalence of Type 2 diabetes in Americans has escalated exponentially. So, now, more than one-half of the States have a prevalence of childhood obesity of greater than 20% of the population.

COST OF OBESITY

The Surgeon General's Report estimated the costs of obesity to be $200 billion each year. One-half of this money is spent on treating the complications of diabetes or other conditions produced by diabetes, such as heart attacks, stroke, kidney failure, and blindness. We hear so much about the detrimental effects of smoking and drinking, but diabetes outranks both of these in its deteriorating effects on health.

COMPLICATIONS OF DIABETES

- Heart attacks
- Strokes
- Renal failure
- Retinopathy (blindness)
- Neuropathy (nerve damage)

TYPE 2 DIABETES

Type 2 diabetes can be prevented or reversed by weight reduction and lifestyle modification. Remarkably, it is frequently cured in those who undergo obesity surgery. Obesity surgery also greatly improves syndrome X and other problems associated with it, namely high cholesterol and high blood pressure.

THE SUGAR-INSULIN RELATIONSHIP

Insulin production, utilization, and storage are the keys to diabetes, which allow sugars to enter the cell and provide energy. When the lock is faulty, sugars cannot enter the cells. As a result, they build up in the bloodstream, where they cause damage.

Carrying excess fat adds to the difficulty that insulin has in doing its job. If the sugar cannot enter the cells, the pancreas goes on pumping out increased insulin in response to the high blood sugar concentration. The insulin may overshoot the mark and produce a rapid fall in blood sugar, which causes powerful appetite stimulation.

INSULIN

- A hormone secreted by the pancreas.
- Permits sugar to enter the cell.
- Controls energy.
- Too little causes diabetes and high blood sugar.
- Too much can lead to a coma.
- Stimulates appetite.
- Converts carbohydrates into fat particles.

Diabetics whose blood sugar is poorly controlled are continuously pouring out excess insulin, to which they become increasingly resistant. The higher levels of blood sugar damage other organs, in particular the eye and the kidney, leading to blindness and renal failure. Extremes of blood sugar concentrations, both low and high, may lead to coma, which is life-threatening. Diabetics also develop accelerated arteriosclerosis, which poses a serious risk of heart attacks, strokes, and gangrene.

GLUCAGON

A second important hormone, "glucagon," which is secreted by the pancreas, acts, in many ways, as an opposite to insulin. Glucagon is released by a protein stimulus, not glucose. Glucagon promotes the mobilization of previously stored fat. So, you tend to burn body fat in response to this hormone rather than storing it in response to insulin.

Carbohydrate-rich meals suppress glucagon secretion. The continued excessive stimulus to insulin production created by the high carbohydrate diet produces insulin resistance. This is, in fact, a diminished effect of insulin in response to more sugar.

REFINED CARBOHYDRATES

Ancient peoples, for many thousands of years, ate unrefined carbohydrates as part of the hunter-gatherer type of diet. With these diets, the pancreas was stimulated to a much lesser extent than with current diets.

Until two hundred years ago, humans ate less than 1 pound of refined sugar per year; now, as stated, 150 pounds are eaten per year. Sugar manufacturers, cola producers, and the packaged food industry have paved the way to the current situation. However cynical it may sound, the sugar manufacturers have contributed to the deaths of more Americans than all wars combined.

GLUCOSE

We eat carbohydrates in the form of simple sugars and starches. All carbohydrates are eventually broken down to the simple sugar glucose. Glucose maintains the blood sugar at a steady level in the nondiabetic. Lesser amounts (600 grams) are stored in the liver and, to a lesser extent, in muscle. Any remaining glucose is converted to and stored as fat.

STARCHES

Complex starches like those found in vegetables are absorbed less rapidly and are slowly broken down to glucose. It is the rapid absorption of ingested refined carbohydrates that increases the blood sugar concentration and stimulates insulin secretion.

BLOOD SUGAR

- Remains stable in normal individuals.
- Increases in the diabetic.
- Stimulates the release of insulin.
- Glucagon counteracts the effect of insulin.
- EXCESS SUGAR CONSUMPTION PRODUCES INSULIN RESISTANCE.

Normal people secrete about 25 to 30 units of insulin per day. Insulin sweeps glucose into the cells where it is stored. Insulin prevents the level of glucose in the blood from rising. Conversely, glucagon in the fasting state prevents the blood sugar from falling too low. Too much insulin can produce dangerously low levels of blood sugar.

As one gains weight, the body's insulin becomes less effective, and more has to be released from the pancreas to reduce blood glucose concentrations. As this advances, the pancreas can't keep up with insulin production. Excessive glucose intake over time, therefore, produces insulin resistance. Then, there is a decreased responsiveness to insulin. This is where fat cells, liver cells, and muscle cells become insensitive to insulin, and blood glucose concentrations rise.

Insulin resistance is a primary factor in the development of obesity. The elevated levels of circulating insulin cause the body to continually store as much fat as possible. Insulin resistance is also the fundamental problem underlying syndrome X. Reducing the intake of sugar will lower the peak insulin levels and reduce insulin resistance.

The precise reasons why insulin resistance occurs are not fully known. Insulin resistance can run in families and is made worse by unhealthy lifestyle habits. These habits are a lack of exercise, poor diet with both nutritional deficiencies and excesses, and substance abuse, together with smoking and drinking.

FAT CHOLESTEROL AND ARTERIOSCLEROSIS

One of the roles of insulin is to convert carbohydrates into minute fat particles called triglycerides. This predisposes us to fat storage, obesity, and, ultimately, heart disease. Triglyceride and cholesterol concentrations in the blood are the main predictive factors for arteriosclerosis. There are two types of cholesterol: high-density lipoprotein (HDL) and low-density lipoprotein (LDL) cholesterol.

In the simplest of terms, high-density lipoprotein cholesterol is good cholesterol, and low-density lipoprotein cholesterol is bad cholesterol. The process of arteriosclerosis, or hardening of the arteries, begins with the development of streaks or plaques of cholesterol on the lining of blood vessels.

Subsequently, these plaques become raised and hard, ultimately leading to “thrombosis” or blockage of the artery. If this occurs in the coronary arteries, it produces angina, a tight, severe pain in the chest, sometimes radiating to the neck and down the arms, which is often produced by exercise. The pain results from a lack of blood supply to the muscles of the heart. The coronary arteries may become completely occluded. This is a condition known as coronary thrombosis. This, in turn, cuts off the blood supply to the heart muscle and leads to death of the muscle fed by that vessel, or myocardial infarction. The most predictive factor for arteriosclerosis is "hyperinsulinism."

ARTERIOSCLEROSIS

- Streaks or plaques of cholesterol are deposited on arterial walls.
- Plaques become raised and hard.
- Clots can develop on the plaques.
- This produces thrombosis.
- Vessel blockage produces gangrene and cell death.

HYPERTENSION

Another problem associated with hyperinsulinism and high blood glucose levels is hypertension, or high blood pressure, also part of syndrome X. Most cases of hypertension are attributed to hyperinsulinism, and this usually precedes the overt diabetic state. Hypertension, in itself, predisposes us to coronary artery disease, stroke, and kidney failure. And it is also a fundamental cause of the main killers of the present day, outlined above.

GOOD FATS AND BAD FATS

For many years, the message about the ill effects of ingested fat prevailed. Fifty years ago, the main villain, in terms of producing the rapidly increasing wave of heart attacks and strokes, was thought to be animal fat. There is, however, now an increasing amount of evidence that unsaturated non-trans fats are good for us. These are not necessarily the fats in margarine; they are fats like olive oil.

THE OMEGA FATTY ACIDS

It has long been known that Mediterranean races have a much lower incidence of coronary artery disease and stroke than Northern Europeans. This may be related to a diet rich in unsaturated fats, which contain omega-3 fatty acids.

A commonly quoted study, the *Lyons Heart Study*, looked at a butter substitute, "canola oil," which is mostly a monounsaturated fat with omega-3 fatty acids. In a series of patients, all of whom had previously had a heart attack, there was a 70% decrease in subsequent heart attacks in those who received the good fat.

Another study, the *GISSI-Prevenzione trial*, showed that fish oil, which contains omega-3 fatty acids, decreased sudden deaths. Omega-3 fatty acids, plentiful in fish, seem to confer some protection against the development of heart attacks and strokes.

Capsules of omega-3 fatty acids in large doses are also effective in treating depressive illnesses. Additionally, a number of studies have shown that nuts, which contain a lot of unsaturated fats, are protective against heart attacks and strokes.

Good fats are called essential fatty acids, which fall into two main categories: the omega-3 and the omega-6 groups. Omega-3 fatty acids are found in leaves and plant seeds, in egg yolks, and in salmon, herring, tuna, and mackerel. Omega-6 fatty acids are found in plant seeds, especially black currants. There are also omega-9 fatty acids, the most plentiful of which, "oleic acid," is found in olive oil, some nuts, and avocados.

The American Heart Association has for many years stated that eating saturated fats such as butter and lard will accelerate the process of arteriosclerosis and lead to the clogging of arteries. Conversely, eating foods high in polyunsaturated fats was thought to keep the arteries clear.

On the other hand, Robert Atkins came out in strong defiance of the dictum; other investigations, including the famous long-standing and most often quoted study, the Framingham Study, realized there was uncertainty surrounding this stance and no factual evidence for its harmfulness.

Supporting Atkins' position, Cestelli has stated, "We found that the people who ate the most cholesterol, or the most saturated fat, or the most calories from fat, weighed the least and were physically the most active."

The combined evidence to date raises fundamental questions about the role of dietary saturated fats in causing heart disease and the supposed role of polyunsaturated fatty acids in preventing it. We need to stick with the philosophy of sugar as being the main enemy.

BALANCING THE FATS

Healthy fat intake certainly depends upon getting the correct proportions of the various fats in the diet. The modern American diet has led to a serious imbalance in the ratio of omega-3 to omega-6 fatty acids. This is a result of consuming a lot of refined corn, soy, sunflower, and canola oils.

It contains copious amounts of omega-6 fatty acids and relatively lesser amounts of omega-3 fatty acids. In contrast, for centuries, the source of essential fatty acids was omega-3-rich whole grains, berries, nuts, vegetables, and egg yolks.

DIET, RACE, AND HEART DISEASE

Native Greenlanders have lived traditionally on a diet that consists of meat and blubber from seals and whales. These mammals feed on fish whose flesh has a high concentration of omega-3 fatty acids. Omega-3 fatty acids lower triglycerides and LDL cholesterol.

Furthermore, they lower blood pressure and have an anticoagulant effect, thus preventing coronary artery thrombosis and stroke. Heart disease is extremely rare in the classical Indigenous Greenland native. Several studies have shown that eating fish reduces death from heart disease.

ALCOHOL

Alcohol, at 8 calories per gram, is rich in energy. Most diets ban alcohol, but alcohol appears to be good for longevity in wine-producing and consuming countries. A glass of wine has fewer calories than a slice of white bread. Beer is widely seen as bad news for anyone counting calories; maltose adds to carbohydrate calories. Beer sales have declined slightly in recent years, while the sales of spirits have increased by 3% per year.

Calories absorbed from alcohol are readily available for utilization as energy. Therefore, they may block fat consumption. Alcohol may also function as an appetite stimulant. In terms of calorie intake, the liquor is not always the problem; it is the soda mixer that goes with it that carries the calories.

Stores are now beginning to sell products like low-carbohydrate mixes, and bars are stocking more diet sodas. Low-carbohydrate and alcohol-free beers are also proliferating, and their taste has greatly improved, making it sometimes difficult to differentiate non-alcoholic from true beer.

- Eight calories per gram.
- Red wine is acceptable.
- Beer is contraindicated as it has a high glycemic index.
- A bottle of spirits contains two days' supply of calories.

CHAPTER 4: THE LONG-TERM HAZARDS OF OBESITY

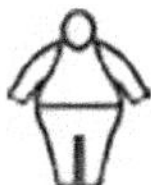

REDUCED LIFE EXPECTANCY

It has been known since the 1950s that men between the ages of 30 and 39 had a progressive increase in mortality due to increasing weight. The increase began with weights just in excess of the acceptable normal weight range. Overall mortality in obese men increases with age thereafter.

Excess weight gain in females is also associated with increased mortality, which begins at an older age than in men. Those overweight men and women who lose substantial amounts of weight and remain at a weight within the optimal range for an appreciable period of time appear to have a lower mortality risk than an equivalent group of overweight individuals. This adds further evidence to the conclusion that obesity decreases lifespan.

The other measurable factor that has a significant influence on longevity is smoking. In non-smoking men and women, the risk of being 35 to 50% overweight, respectively, confers the same risk as smoking with a body weight within the acceptable range.

Obesity has been shown to have a significant role to play in the genesis of coronary artery disease. There are, however, other strong risk factors, including age, male sex, hypertension, smoking, and elevated cholesterol concentrations.

Some of these other risk factors, particularly high blood pressure and serum cholesterol, are directly related to obesity. Another factor related to heart disease and obesity is physical inactivity. This has been scientifically shown in many studies to be related to the development of heart disease. It plays a role in obesity at all ages. It has been shown that both vigorous exercise and walking are protective not only from the point of view of preventing the development of obesity but also from coronary artery disease. The exact mechanism of the protective effect is not fully understood.

Studies on the role of blood pressure and the relationship between blood pressure and obesity are somewhat conflicting. However, there is good evidence that as weight increases with age, there is an elevation in blood pressure. This is mainly because the heart has to pump blood around a significant excess of body tissue in the circulation, which increases the resistance to flow.

RISKS OF OBESITY

- Heart attack
- Hypertension
- Stroke
- High cholesterol levels
- Diabetes
- Gallstones
- Gout
- Osteoarthritis
- Kidney stones
- Cancer: breast, uterus, cervix

STONE FORMATION

Kidney and gallstone formation are also closely related to obesity. Gallstones probably result from the ingestion of excessive amounts of cholesterol and changes in liver function, which deposit more cholesterol in the bile of the obese subject.

Another factor that predisposes to gallstone formation in the obese is the use of inappropriate crash-slimming diets. Rapid reductions in weight or prolonged periods of starvation undoubtedly, conversely, predispose toward the development of gallstones.

JOINT DISEASES

Gout is a complication of obesity, the probability of which increases in those who are over 30% of their appropriate weight. Sufferers from gout develop uric acid stones in their kidneys. Osteoarthritis is a common condition that occurs progressively with increasing weight. This is a wear and tear process of the cartilage that lines joints, producing erosion and damage to the joint space with exposure of bone to bone within the joint.

Usually, it occurs as a result of damage to the joints that are most vulnerable to the obese state, in particular, the hips and knee joints. Arthritis produces joint pain and restricts exercise tolerance, thus creating a vicious circle leading to further weight gain.

CANCER

The American Cancer Society has shown an association between obesity and increased risk of cancers of the colon, rectum, and prostate. With increasing weight, women show a progressive increase in the risk of cancer of the breast, uterus, and cervix.

HEART AND LUNG DISEASE

Obesity places a considerable burden on the heart and respiratory systems. Lung function becomes increasingly impaired with increasing weight. It further impairs exercise tolerance. Ultimately, the morbidly obese patient with a combination of heart, lung, and joint disease becomes beleaguered and totally unable to perform any form of exercise. Even walking or climbing stairs becomes severely restricted.

Another common problem associated with obesity is "sleep apnea." Sleep apnea is a condition in which levels of oxygen within the bloodstream fall during sleep, leading to sleep fragmentation, frequent awakening, and the development of right-sided heart failure. This is associated with maladies of brain function. This may occur as a result of damage to the central nervous system. The course of this condition is chronic and progressive; it is, however, reversible by weight loss.

TOBACCO

People who smoke cigarettes are significantly lighter than nonsmokers. Differences are greatest in the lower socioeconomic groups. It is well documented that body weight increases when smokers give up their habit. And this, unfortunately, is often used by smokers as a reason to persist in their habit. While smoking is an appetite suppressant, the explanation for the weight gain that occurs when smoking is stopped may be related to an increase in energy intake or a fall in energy expenditure.

Smokers who give up the habit are particularly prone to take sweets and snacks. These are considered to form a substitute for cigarettes. It is also considered that cigarette smoking increases the metabolic rate, possibly by stimulating the sympathetic nervous system with nicotine. When the balance between obesity and smoking is considered, there is no doubt that smoking is more damaging than being overweight. And there is nothing worse for your health than smoking.

LONG-TERM HAZARDS OF OBESITY

- Shortened life expectancy
- Diabetes mellitus
- Coronary artery disease
- Renal failure
- Heart failure
- Respiratory failure
- Liver failure
- Stroke
- Osteoarthritis of the hips and knees
- Gallstones
- Sleep apnea
- Kidney stones
- Deep vein thrombosis
- Pulmonary hypertension
- Dermatological problems
- Cellulitis
- Infections and septicemia
- Cancer of the colon, rectum, prostate, breast, uterus, and cervix

CHAPTER 5: THE FUTURE—A POTENTIAL DECLINE IN LIFE EXPECTANCY AS A RESULT OF OBESITY

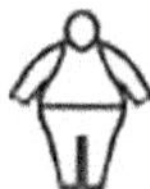

Forecasts of life expectancy form a critical component of government strategy with regard to such programs as "Social Security" and "Medicare." Until recently, all forecasts of life expectancy favored a continuing increase.

For the past one thousand years, there has been a slow and steady increase in life expectancy, occasionally punctuated by epidemics, famines, and major wars. The risk of major pandemics declined after the influenza outbreak at the end of World War I, which killed more people than the war. This was, however, virtually superseded by the COVID-19 pandemic of 2020. And potentially, more pandemics could be on the way! These pandemics could principally annihilate the elderly population.

Gains in life expectancy at older ages are now much smaller than they were in the first half of the 20th century, and they may now have begun to decline. Some prognostications of life expectancy have been overly optimistic.

The United Nations forecasts a projected life expectancy of one hundred years for males and females in developed countries by the year 2030. The Social Security Administration arrived at a figure of life expectancy reaching the mid-eighties later this century; these figures are now somewhat questionable.

THE LIFE-SHORTENING EFFECT OF OBESITY

The above forecasts are now seriously being questioned as a result of the unprecedented increase in obesity in the United States and the risk of further pandemics. If current trends continue, these will undoubtedly threaten to diminish the health and life expectancy of current and future generations. As has been stated, two-thirds of adults in the United States today are obese or overweight, and 70% of African Americans are currently obese.

As stated in an article in the *New England Journal of Medicine*, children and ethnic minorities have shown the greatest increase in obesity. These trends have affected all major racial and ethnic groups and all socioeconomic strata. It is now estimated that obesity causes over a quarter of a million deaths per year in the United States. The risk of developing diabetes in the United States has risen exponentially to between 30 and 40%. If the prevalence of obesity continues to rise, it will lead to an elevated risk of associated morbidities with a negative effect on longevity.

Obesity reduces life expectancy by between 5 and 20 years, averaging 13 years. And this increases with increasing excess weight. A continued rise in the prevalence of obesity could, for the first time in one thousand years, lead to a statistical downturn in longevity for the whole population.

OTHER THREATS TO INCREASED LONGEVITY

There are other realistic threats to increases in life expectancy, such as an increase in viral epidemics, the development of new infectious diseases that are resistant to antibiotics, and the emergence of aggressive new strains of viruses such as the influenza virus—the latest variant of which is referred to as the "bird flu."

In addition, there has been the devastating effect produced by COVID-19, whose exact origins are still open to worldwide debate. Infectious diseases have, over the centuries, always presented the greatest threat to life expectancy. Another major threat has been famine, which still exists in relation to warfare. But now, for the first time, the major and inevitable threat to increased longevity relates directly to the presence of obesity in today's society.

CHAPTER 6: THE BASIC CAUSES OF OBESITY

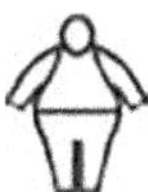

Why do people become excessively obese? The essential answer is that, in the long term, they ingest calories significantly in excess of their needs. It has been shown that the obese inherit a lower metabolic rate than normal-weight individuals. But as they gain weight, the metabolic rate goes up to compensate and provide energy for the maintenance of their excess weight.

- Q—why do people become obese?
- A—because they consistently take in more calories than they burn. There is an easy answer.
- Q—why is obesity becoming so common?
- A—because of lifestyle changes, eating the wrong food, sitting in front of computers and televisions, being influenced by food advertisements, and taking no action.

OBESITY IS NOT GENETIC—IT IS BEHAVIORAL

Obesity often begins early in life; there has been a doubling in the incidence of obesity in three and four-year-old children in the last decade. During this time, there has been no change in birth weight and no change in the gene pool. Thus, obesity in children is acquired and relates primarily to lifestyle!

Factors that contribute to this are the increased consumption of fast food and high-calorie carbohydrate drinks, reduced physical activity brought on by the use of social media, food advertising, and less breastfeeding. These factors are strongly influenced by parental control.

THE POWER OF ADVERTISING

Advertising is a powerful factor in the vicious equation. Food marketers target children and adults to influence their food choices and eating behavior. So lucrative is this business that large companies contract to provide free computers and televisions to schools in exchange for compelling the children to view two minutes of commercial messages each day.

Food advertising makes up a considerable proportion of this viewing time. This reflects on the way in which the nation's schools are funded. In relative terms, education has become increasingly poorly financed. Furthermore, the effects of the advertising campaigns are surreptitious and difficult to evaluate, but they can be overwhelming.

We are all immersed in a sea of advertising to a much greater extent than we are aware. If advertising were not so influential, companies would not invest in it. But observation of the plethora of advertising on television, the internet, in the press, and on our streets only emphasizes its relevance.

SCHOOLS—STARTING ON THE WRONG TRACK

In the past decade, in some school districts, fast food companies took over school food service operations. Under these circumstances, the fast-food company eliminates the burden on the school of providing meals that the child will eat. The question of appropriate nutrition, physical activity, and weight management never entered the equation. These meal services are often supplemented by vending machines, which provide an endless supply of sugar. This is again accessible throughout the day.

At the end of the last century, these sales to school distributors increased by 1100%. Each can of soda contains the equivalent of ten teaspoons of sugar. One large soda drink can supply one-half of the total daily caloric count required by a teenager. The average child consumes in excess of one can of soda per day. A correlation exists between soda consumption and obesity in childhood. Soda consumption combined with an increasing lack of exercise is a potent combination in the production of obesity.

The above social factors driving obesity in childhood have been generated by and are equally present in adults. As stated, adults walk less, drive more cars, and use more public transport than ever before. There are more elevators, escalators, conveyor belts, televisions, computers, and more couches.

Conversely, there are more gymnasiums, sales of exercise equipment, jogging tracks, and other sports facilities. The latter, however, are only used by a small, preselected cross-section of the community. However, because of the physical encumbrance produced by their excess fat, morbidly obese patients cannot use these aids.

EXCESS ENERGY INTAKE

The exact mechanism by which man controls his energy intake in order to maintain a steady weight is unknown. A "set point" seems to exist. This, in practical terms, is a buffer zone around which most people keep their weight fairly constant.

THE SET POINT

- A point of stability around which the body weight remains stable.

- Consistently eating more calories than are burned raises the set point.
- Once elevated, it is very difficult to get down again.
- It is a buffer zone for weight.

Factors affecting this set point are satiety—a feeling of adequate food intake; neurohumoral factors; distention of the stomach; and the effects of stimulating the nerve fibers between the stomach and the brain. In trying to maintain the set point, the body intrinsically tries to control its calorie intake; increased intake, up to a point, stimulates activity.

Whereas decreased intake tends to reduce physical activity through an expression of tiredness or the induction of a restful state. It is possible for the body to reset the set point in an upward direction so that prolonged and continuous excess food intake produces elevation of the point of equilibrium. Conversely, the defense of the set point has been used to explain why the maintenance of medically induced weight loss has been so poor.

ENERGY CONSERVATION: THE MODE

Energy conservation is a factor that influences short-term weight stability. So, often, one hears from patients that they have virtually starved for a few days and have not lost any weight. When fasting (conservation mode), the body probably reduces energy output by reducing the metabolic rate to compensate for the sudden close-off of food intake. This is probably not only confined to metabolic rate but also to energy usage by the body for exercise and day-to-day activities. Such conservation is probably related to the set point.

ENERGY EXPENDITURE

- Basal metabolic rate: 1200 cal
- Walking: 250 calories per hour

- Cycling: 350 calories per hour
- Running: 400 to 600 calories per hour

THE AUTONOMIC NERVOUS SYSTEM

Energy expenditure is influenced to a large extent by activity generated by the sympathetic nervous system. The sympathetic nervous system may be likened to an electrical system of wiring that is distributed throughout the whole body. Its function is often illustrated by stating that it is the system by which our body responds to "fright, fight, and flight."

In other words, it is a system of physical activation. The chemicals that act as transmitters in the sympathetic nervous system are adrenaline and related compounds. The functional counterpoint to the sympathetic nervous system is called the parasympathetic system; its electrical pathways mainly run through the vagus nerve, a nerve that runs from the hypothalamus in the brain to the heart, lungs, and intestines.

The hypothalamus, part of the base of the brain, is functionally intimately related to appetite. Destruction of one area of the hypothalamus increases vagus nerve firing (parasympathetic) and decreases sympathetic activity. Stimulation of the vagus nerve triggers pancreatic insulin release and makes the stomach empty at a faster rate, thus promoting obesity.

Congenital abnormalities of the hypothalamus, such as the Prader-Willi syndrome, are associated with a morbidly obese state. In addition to factors that stimulate the parasympathetic nervous system, anything that inhibits sympathetic activity leads to weight gain. Different areas in the hypothalamus have differing effects on appetite; there is an area at the front and on the outside of the hypothalamus. This, when damaged, causes a reduction in food intake and an increase in energy expenditure.

Neurosurgeons have attempted to treat obesity by damaging this critical area in the brain. Studies of autonomic nervous system function have found that obese patients have a depression of both sympathetic and parasympathetic activity.

HORMONAL FACTORS—THYROID HORMONE

Many who suffer from obesity feel that their underlying problem is hormonal or "glandular" and that the thyroid gland, in particular, is the source of the problem. There is no evidence that obese patients have a different thyroid level of hormonal response to changes in energy than normal non-obese individuals.

Under the activity of the thyroid gland, a condition called "myxedema" will predispose to obesity, just as the overactive state of thyrotoxicosis is associated with weight loss and increased sympathetic activity. It is for this reason that many have attempted to use thyroid hormone for the treatment of obesity.

Increased levels of thyroid hormones increase the patient's metabolic rate and may also produce undesirable and potentially dangerous complications such as cardiac rhythmic disturbances. This may lead to cardiac failure or even sudden death. Anxiety, tremors, sweating, or palpitations are other side effects of the use of thyroid hormone. Where thyroxine has been used in the treatment of obesity, the results have been unimpressive.

CORTICOSTEROIDS

Cushing's syndrome—which occurs due to excessive production of corticosteroids by the adrenal gland—may produce obesity. However, the condition is distinctly uncommon and rarely contributes to the problem in the obese patient. Adrenalectomy in animals has been associated with weight loss.

CUSHING'S SYNDROME

- Central obesity
- Buffalo hump
- Peripheral purple striae
- Muscle wasting
- Hypertension
- Peptic ulceration

Sex Hormones

Sex hormones influence the accumulation and distribution of fat. Females, on the whole, have a higher percentage of body fat than males. And most morbidly obese people are female. The distribution of fat is also different between the sexes. Males deposit fat on the central abdomen and become "pot-bellied." Females concentrate the fat on the lower abdomen, buttocks, and thighs, becoming "pear-shaped."

Growth Hormone

Growth hormone has been advocated for use in weight loss programs and is also used in an attempt to preserve male strength and prevent aging. The use of growth hormones does not alter body habitus by redistributing fat and promoting muscle growth.

- Excess growth hormone produces:
- Acromegaly
- Large size-gigantism
- Strong muscles
- Large hands
- Large jaw
- Brain tumors can also produce this.

GUT HORMONES

The gut produces many hormones, often with variable action and interdependence; most of these decrease food intake. These hormones affect the secretion of acid and pancreatic juice; some have an influence on the motility or contraction of the intestines. There is no real evidence that any of the hormones, under normal circumstances, play a significant role in the problem of obesity.

Below are listed some of the naturally occurring chemicals that may affect the obese state:

- Leptin
- Resistin
- Neuropeptide Y
- C-75
- Ghrelin

There have been several recent important observations that might assist in our understanding of the cause and treatment of obesity.

GHRELIN

In contrast to other gut hormones, a recently discovered substance, ghrelin, increases food intake. Ghrelin, which is produced by the stomach, stimulates growth hormone release and causes excessive eating and obesity in rats. Levels of this hormone are, on the whole, lower in obese subjects. However, they do not decrease after a meal, as they do in subjects of normal weight.

Interestingly, levels of ghrelin in the body may increase after dieting, but are decreased by obesity surgery. This might, therefore, be a factor influencing the weight loss that occurs after surgery. Ghrelin sends a signal to the brain to eat whenever the stomach is empty and to slow down when it is full. Some patients are now being experimentally treated with electronic pacemakers that apparently have a ghrelin-like effect, convincing the stomach that it is fuller than it actually is.

Ghrelin from the stomach tells the brain it is time to eat. Cholecystokinin tells the brain it's time to stop eating. Leptin and insulin are stimulating factors that help to maintain the set point.

C-75

This substance, when administered to mice, reduced food intake by 90%. C-75-treated mice lost 45% more weight than totally fasting animals. This occurred because C-75 inhibits feeding but does not decrease the metabolic rate or energy expenditure, as does fasting.

NEUROPEPTIDE-Y

Neuropeptide-Y is a naturally occurring substance in the brain that, when directly introduced into the brains of animals, produces voracious feeding. It is the most powerful appetite stimulant known. The substance inhibits thermogenesis, the heat generated by burning calories. During starvation, neuropeptide-Y levels increase. Levels of insulin fall during starvation and may help to stimulate a rise in neuropeptide-Y.

The action of neuropeptide-Y, which is completely blocked by C-75, is independent of leptin (vide infra). Neuropeptide-Y suppresses the sympathetic nervous system and produces marked weight gain in animals. The effects of this substance are mediated through a specific receptor in the brain, the so-called Y-receptor. There have been several recent important observations that could assist in our understanding of the cause and treatment of weight loss.

LEPTIN

Leptin is one of half a dozen or so chemical messengers produced by and stored in fat cells. These include clotting agents, blood vessel constricting agents, and inflammatory agents that have powerful effects throughout the body.

Leptin is a protein gene that is defective in obese mice and obese humans. There is some evidence to suggest that the replacement of leptin reverses obesity in animals. Studies in humans have been disappointing in their outcome. Leptin is thought to signal adequacy of food intake, but high levels do little to burn off the stimulus to eat. When leptin was injected into mice, they suddenly changed their eating habits and began shedding fat. All mice have the leptin gene, but unfortunately, it exists in only a handful of people.

In those with the gene, it has been shown to produce dramatic weight loss. In those that do not have the gene, it is pretty well ineffective. Some of the compounds discussed above, like C-75 and neuropeptide-Y, would, on theoretical grounds, at the present time, seem to offer more promise of a future therapeutic role than leptin. C-75 is a synthetic derivative of a naturally occurring substance called cerulenin.

RESISTIN

The hormone "resistin" was discovered at the turn of the century. This is a resistance to the insulin hormone, and is a protein molecule found in fat cells. The hormone is elevated in obesity and in insulin-resistant patients. When fat cells are replete, they release resistin, and insulin resistance ensues. However, the hormone is decreased in rodent obesity models and paradoxically increased by insulin-sensitizing drugs. A group of drugs, the thiazolidinediones, suppress the expression of resistin.

OREXINS AND MELANIN-STIMULATING HORMONE

Orexins are substances found in the hypothalamus that increase food intake. In contrast, the substance melanocyte-stimulating hormone from the pituitary gland inhibits food intake and results in weight loss.

FAT STORAGE

Fat storage evolved over millions of years as the primary mechanism for coping with periods of famine. For most of the period of evolution, the major problem was getting enough to eat in order to survive the winter rather than avoiding obesity. When calorie intake exceeds expenditure, fat cells swell to as much as six times their minimum size, and they begin to multiply.

In the average adult, there is something of the order of 40 billion fat cells, which can increase up to 100 billion. Losing weight causes the fat cells to shrink in size and become less metabolically active. However, their number goes down only very slowly, if at all.

FAT CELLS, INFLAMMATION, AND IMMUNITY

The process of inflammation is currently receiving a lot of attention. Fat cells promote inflammation, which can spread throughout the body. Even small amounts of excess fat can produce a mounting immune response. This is largely because the body regards the storage of excess fat cells as an invading organism and attempts to reject it by mounting an inflammatory response.

Inflammation is now viewed as a key mechanism in heart disease, probably being more important than cholesterol per se. Blood vessels such as the coronary arteries are undoubtedly narrowed by cholesterol. But a big problem appears to be that an inflamed plaque can break open, produce a clot, and occlude a vessel—a process known as thrombosis.

In the case of the coronary arteries, this leads to the death of the heart muscle. Compounds secreted by fat cells contribute to vascular inflammation. They inhibit nitric oxide, a compound that helps relax blood vessel walls and lowers blood pressure. Fat cells also secrete estrogen. This is linked to certain types of cancer and obesity.

Researchers now suspect that the origin of diabetes lies, at least partly, in the biochemistry of fat, in particular in compounds made by fat cells. These are resistin and tumor necrosis factor. Resistin promotes the conversion of fatty acids into glucose by the liver, a process that is useful during starvation but a potential hazard in obese patients. The amount of resistance that the body produces increases with the amount of fat stored. Tumor necrosis factor, a naturally occurring substance, promotes insulin resistance.

Fat cells behave differently in different parts of the body. Fat carried in the hips and thighs is considered comparatively benign, whereas that which accumulates around the organs in the abdomen is more harmful. The latter is more metabolically active and produces more inflammation and clot-promoting compounds than does fat distributed around the periphery of the body.

Fortunately, visceral fat is the first to disappear in response to exercise, a key point in favor of regular exercise. The actual distribution of body fat is genetically determined. However, the amount of fat stored relates directly to the excess intake of calories over output.

OBESITY GENES

Obesity genes have been identified, but their role is ill-defined. The overall balance between energy intake and expenditure is pretty finely tuned, and only small deviations on a daily basis can produce changes in weight. A 1% excess of intake over expenditure stored as fat would produce a weight gain of 1.25 kg in one year.

Achieving this very accurate balance depends upon an extremely complex interaction of hormonal activity, temperature exposure, the set point, and other factors. The major role of hormones is that ghrelin, produced by the stomach, tells the brain it is time to eat. When food leaves the stomach, another hormone, "cholecystokinin," is released. This signals that the meal is over and triggers the release of other enzymes important for the digestion of proteins, carbohydrates, and fats. Leptin and insulin are our longer-term stabilizing factors that influence fat deposits.

All of the above factors act in concert to maintain the "set point." C-75 could lower the set point. Eating too many refined carbohydrates or too much fried food can affect the delicate balance by interfering with the action of leptin and insulin in the brain. The appetite center in the hypothalamus is also affected by a number of drugs and alcohol. Genetic variation can also push people to eat more food, but obesity is, by and large, a behavioral problem.

CHAPTER 7: THE TECHNOLOGICAL REVOLUTION

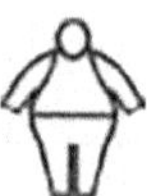

Modern humans developed between 100,000 and 150,000 years ago, coincidentally with the invention of controlled agriculture. A steady and predictable source of food, which could be replenished through the seasons, led to the development of large population centers. The shift from wild meat and vegetation to cultivated grains deprived humans of many of the essential amino acids, vitamins, and minerals that they had thrived on for millions of years. Although lifespan increased, average height diminished, and nutritional problems began to accrue.

Nutritional deficiencies started to manifest themselves in skeletal remains, dental cavity development, and an increase in bacterial infections. Obesity, however, was not a problem. This remained the situation until approximately 100 years ago, when the technological revolution led to a reduced need for hard physical labor.

Improved technology has made crops of grain and dairy products both cheaper to produce and much more plentiful. Along with these changes has come the bubble of obesity. This could result in a reduction in life expectancy for the first time in centuries. The explosion in the prevalence of obesity is related to socioeconomic changes.

SOCIOECONOMICS OF OBESITY

In the United States, wealthy people tend to be thinner than those of lower socioeconomic status. One in four adults living below the poverty line is obese, compared with one in six in households with an income in excess of $70,000 per year. In addition, one in three African Americans is obese.

SOCIOECONOMICS AND OBESITY

- Fast foods are inexpensive, readily available, and eaten quickly.
- Carbohydrates are less expensive than protein.
- Eating well is expensive.
- In restaurants, the cheaper the food, the less healthy it is.
- Higher-income individuals tend to be slimmer.

The reasons for the above are not altogether clear. It does not appear to be a simple question of eating sweet cakes instead of crispy greens. Processed foods are not just cheap; they are tasty and filling. Calorically, the best value for money is a food high in refined sugar content. Lean fish or steak is much more expensive than hamburgers.

Children, particularly, are prone to eating the wrong foods. They have some money but not a lot, and their parents are out at work. Consequently, they go to the corner store and buy junk food. They eat this before the television sets on which these colorful and tasty products have been attractively advertised.

The power of advertising cannot be underestimated. One of the implications of this has been the provision of large portions of food. In the running of a restaurant, only about 20% of the retail price goes toward food. Therefore, it is not expensive to increase the amount of food given to the consumer.

Advertising supersized meals at a bargain price is a major factor in successful marketing. Unfortunately, it results in overeating with stretching of the stomach and, subsequently, the desire to eat more with each meal; this then becomes a habit. A vicious cycle develops so that, ultimately, the consumer, whether in a restaurant or at home, becomes used to taking much larger meals.

Portion size increase can result in a rise in caloric intake of anything from 300 to 500 calories with each meal. Along with the "bargain binge" has gone a markedly increased tendency to eat in restaurants. Approximately 50% of food budgets are now spent in restaurants. Here, in order to make the supersized meals tastier and more attractive, additional fats and carbohydrates are added. Unfortunately, the kind of fat that is used has a high trans fatty acid concentration.

French fries, bread, pastry, and salad dressing are among the items that contain trans fatty acids. An important factor that has led to more eating out and the consumption of more fast food by children has been the ever-increasing tendency for both parents and the family to be engaged in full-time employment. Under such circumstances, incomes are higher, and the tendency to want to cook after a full day's work is understandably low. The result, therefore, has been to consume fast food in restaurants.

CHAPTER 8: THE PSYCHOLOGY OF THE OBESE STATE

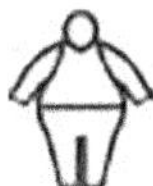

OBESITY AND SELF-ESTEEM

Psychiatric problems are commonly associated with the state of obesity. Whether they are causative of, or consequential to, obesity may be debated. It is hardly surprising that morbidly obese individuals who cannot climb a flight of stairs, sit in a normal seat, buy and wear conventional clothes, or get on the bus or a plane would have low self-esteem.

Low self-esteem leads to social isolation. Many obese patients will not go out of their houses during daylight hours. Social isolation produces depression, and food provides solace to the depressed. Associated physical disorders such as sleep apnea, diabetes, hypertension, and vascular disease can also lead to changes in the psyche. Therefore, a psychiatrist or psychologist needs to be an important member of the ideal management team for the obese subject.

A BEHAVIORAL PROBLEM

It should be observed that the massively increased prevalence of obesity in the past few decades cannot be attributed to either a change in genetics or the onset of recognizable psychiatric disorders. Instead, behavioral, cultural, and submission to extrinsic pressures, such as food advertisements, and a consequence of an acquired aberration of the role and value of nutrients, also serve as major contributors.

Such behavioral influences might lead more people to "live to eat" rather than "eat to live." This naturally indicates addictive behavior, which could be a significant component. Addiction to food is ostensibly more of a problem than addiction to alcohol or drugs.

Why? Because, as difficult as the latter two are to manage, the patient may temporarily be taken away from alcohol or drugs. All the while, food is essential to life! Not only is food essential, but we are what we eat: the accurate balance, as a necessary provider, may be remarkably difficult to control once the homeostatic mechanisms fall away.

The homeostatic mechanisms that regulate eating behavior, present throughout the animal kingdom, are becoming grossly distorted in man for the first time in thousands of years. Throughout history, man has suffered more from the implications of starvation than from a plethora of food. However, gluttony and obesity existed with other excesses in the period of affluence of the Roman era.

Although the ravages of malnutrition and the extreme cases of starvation in Nigeria and other Central African countries are depicted periodically by the media, we may have again entered an era where more suffer from excess than a shortage of food. A remarkable degree of sophistication and control goes into body weight maintenance.

The 20-pound weight gain experienced by the average American between the ages of 25 and 55 years represents a remarkably small net imbalance between energy intake and expenditure. It is equal to an excess intake over expenditure of 0.3% of ingested calories or apparently as little as 6 cal per day!

The average annual food intake is one million calories: 200 pounds of carbohydrate, 66 pounds of fat, and 50 pounds of protein. Numerous biological and psychological influences may modify eating behavior. The hypothalamus, the sympathetic, and parasympathetic nervous systems, discussed previously, are functionally influenced by psychological factors.

Dietary composition per se is not a determinant of body makeup. Since both protein and carbohydrate can be efficiently converted into fat, there is no evidence that changing the relative proportions of protein, carbohydrate, and fat in the diet without reducing overall calorie intake will indeed promote weight loss.

PSYCHOLOGICAL FACTORS

That psychological factors are imperative in governing our caloric intake is clear when we look at studies that attempt to eliminate these factors. A study was carried out where pre-weighed bottles of milk were delivered to the houses of 37 babies. The bottles were then collected for re-weighing and the determination of food intake.

Varying the dilution of the milk, of which the mothers were unaware, was given at different times. The babies fed with half-strength milk increased their volume intake by 80%, but not 100%. This result suggests that appetite may be related to volume rather than energy intake. Later in life, individual food preferences would make such a study impossible.

Studies in older malnourished children in Jamaica, however, demonstrated the development of a voracious appetite after long-term food deprivation. This might be an explanation for the often-observed rapid weight gain that follows a period of extreme dieting.

Outside of infancy, psychological factors soon impose a considerable influence on dietary intake. These factors are affected by the color, texture, smell, taste, and energy content of food. Studies have shown that the individual's selection of food reflects a response to food availability and palatability rather than energy content, hence the effect of fast foods on weight increase.

These factors are social as well as psychological. The situation is complex, as animals may shift their food intake in order to obtain sufficient amounts of the essential minerals or vitamins when food concentrations of the latter are low. If such instincts ever existed in men, they have now probably been lost.

SOCIETY AND EATING HABITS

Societies in various nations have developed an antagonistic attitude toward obesity. Obese children tend to be disliked, looked down upon, and become the subject of offhand jokes. Their obese state is associated with shame, as they are thought to be self-indulgent and lacking in willpower.

Generally, obese children are regarded as being responsible for their condition, whereas disabled children are not, and the latter receive sympathy and support. The feeding of babies and children has substantial emotional overtones, and the provision of food is often associated with signs of affection.

Obese parents tend to beget or create obese children. The availability and palatability of food influence intake. The high caloric value of food tends to equate with palatability. At the same time, foods high in sugar content tend to be more available by being cheaper than more ideal foods.

Social and family pressures can lead to overeating, as it is often regarded as a sign of appreciation to eat the food presented as much as possible. We spend so much time sitting around the table eating. Important life events such as birthdays, successes, marriages, and even funerals are celebrated with a feast. Such practices are not new: the Romans developed great pleasure from eating and often overate in a gluttonous fashion.

"Ear ticklers" existed in Roman times, people who were skilled at rubbing the ears of those who had overeaten. They served this purpose only to induce vomiting and thereby enable the party to go on: to start eating again. The mechanism behind this procedure was that the vagus nerve, or wandering nerve, supplies not only the stomach but also branches to the external ear. Stimulation of the ear activates the vagus nerve and can produce contractions of the stomach, which induce vomiting.

THE RITUAL OF EATING

Eating food becomes an important ritual. We all like good food and its varieties, and we not only socialize around the table but also hold business meetings as well. If indeed food becomes an addiction—which is the case in several morbidly obese individuals—then it is that addiction with which the addicted must contend constantly. Why? Because food is not only essential, but is also always around us.

Diets eaten in different countries vary a lot. However, most nations have, over the centuries, developed diets which, though widely differing in their content, maintain the body in good functional health without any marked nutritional deficiencies. Recently, studies have shown that Puerto Rican women living in the continental United States increase their weight by living there longer. This is persuasive evidence that social factors, rather than genetic ones, are of fundamental importance.

OBESITY AND DEPRESSION

Though difficult to categorize accurately, the psychological factors that pertain to the obese state are significant and considerable. The higher the body mass index, the greater the incidence of depression. A number of factors contribute to the overall development of psychological problems, which culminate in chronic depression.

Discrimination leads to low self-worth and a reduced quality of life. Family and sexual relationships suffer, and problems frequently arise in the workplace. Employment can be difficult to obtain for the morbidly obese.

Over two-thirds of obese patients report abuse, physical in 34%, sexual in 12%, and psychological in 64%. All the while, one-third of obese patients report a family history of alcoholism. Conversely, however, alcoholism is rare in the morbidly obese subject.

BODY IMAGE AND THE PSYCHE

Body image is an important aspect of overall self-image. A woman who was sexually abused in childhood may use her size as a protection against attracting men. Despite her desire to lose weight, she may get more and more anxious as she becomes shapelier. Another person who equates food with love or weight with power will experience immense inner conflict about changing his or her lifestyle when losing weight.

To be successful, all psychotherapy must address emotional dysregulation, impulsive behavior, and cognitive/perceptual distortions. Group and individual therapy, particularly cognitive behavioral therapy, can highlight rationalizations, reframe negative patterns of thinking, and provide a more realistic manner of self-assessment. A recognition of one's own mental functioning and how one solves problems is imperative in reshaping those attitudes from the past, which may sabotage dieting efforts.

FATNESS WAS EQUATED WITH SUCCESS

Early in the 20th century, when tuberculosis and other infectious diseases were still rampant, being thin was often perceived as a sign of sickness, poverty, or neglect. The prize of every family was plump, "healthy" children; the plump female was "womanly." All the while, the plump male, with their watch chains stretched across the waist-coated belly, looked "prosperous." Most people had heard of calories and knew that sweets were fattening, but paid little or no attention to the caloric contents of what they ate.

When World War II brought rationing, meat and butter became luxury items. Gas was rationed, and people walked. Yet, most middle-aged adults in the United States were overweight, and few exercised for health. It was expected that a woman would lose her "figure" after 30 and have to wear a girdle. Men padded their shoulders and wore double-breasted suits to hide middle-aged bellies. Being old was synonymous with being fat, and nobody knew anything that could be done to change the scenario.

THE IMPACT OF TELEVISION

After the war, the biggest change in American life came through television. TV changed the eating habits of America, but not for the better! The "TV dinner" predominated as the American menu since everyone gathered around the new *center* of the home.

Television's advertising potential was quickly realized and exploited by the food industry, telling children to eat more sugary cereal. And also tempting adults to enjoy and indulge in "double cheeseburgers," chips, meats, and multiple snacks.

ADVERTISING OF FOOD

Advertising showed America the face it wanted to see: big, affluent, and carefree, untouched by war or want. Cars were oversized, sporting big fins and capacious seats. In the new supermarkets, myriad food packages promised "*more*" for your money. Restaurants served big steaks on bigger plates, along with the new huge "salad bar." Truly, only too much was enough.

It was no wonder indeed that Americans learned to overeat, long before the crisis of today progressed.

PSYCHOLOGICAL ASPECTS RELATED TO EXERCISE

Lack of exercise is an important factor in the obesity equation. It has been discovered that the less walking a person does in his day-to-day activities, the more likely he is to be overweight. Exercise increases academic performance, assertiveness, confidence, emotional stability, independence, memory, mood, sexual satisfaction, and overall well-being. In addition, exercise programs result in lower rates of absenteeism, anger, anxiety, depression, and even alcohol abuse.

Obese subjects are often opposed to exercise programs. They are self-conscious and frequently have difficulty performing the exercises because they are carrying so much extra weight, or they may be restricted by joint pains or breathlessness.

Many morbidly obese patients are too disabled to exercise or even climb a flight of stairs. Those who can exercise are frequently discouraged by the slow results achieved from exercise programs. And also the fact that a can of cola contains all the calories expended in a 30-minute exercise schedule!

The importance of exercise cannot be overemphasized. Exercise is important from the point of view of preventing heart attacks, strokes, and the development of diabetes. The benefits of exercise are clearly visible in increased muscle mass and often increased activity and alertness.

Exercise does not necessarily increase hunger. As a matter of fact, a 30-to-40-minute walk produces well-being by virtue of an endorphin drive and can lead to a suppression of appetite. Also, the results of participating in an exercise program are a disincentive for the subject to go home and eat excessive amounts of food.

Exercise does burn calories and tends to increase basal metabolic rate, thus giving rise to a further erosion of the calorific load. Another useful manifestation of exercise is that it stimulates muscle production and converts fat into muscle.

Finally, the endorphin drive produced by exercise results in a feeling of well-being and enables people to adapt to a more positive attitude toward life and its problems. Exercise, in itself, however, must be stated, does not greatly contribute to weight loss in the obese patient.

CHAPTER 9: MAJOR EATING DISORDERS

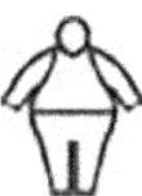

The three major eating disorders are *anorexia nervosa, bulimia nervosa* (bingeing and purging), and *binge eating disorder* (binge eating only). Anorexia nervosa has been well recognized for over 50 years. And its prevalence has increased and continues to increase yearly. However, little is known of the underlying cause as it remains elusive. What's more, nothing has recently been added to its treatment. This is a condition in which a major underlying factor is a fear of being fat and can develop from an early age. The onset of anorexia most frequently occurs during the teenage years. The vast majority of cases are females, but the number of males is now increasing. The condition has the highest mortality rate among all psychiatric disorders.

Eating disorders take control of the individual and become their primary focus in life. Sufferers focus on the specifics of extreme calorie restriction and food avoidance. This is coupled with sometimes excessive exercising, usually walking, which is all they have the strength to do.

Anorexics are terrified of being fat! They binge and purge using self-induced vomiting, laxatives, or excessive exercise to compensate for their loss of eating control. Those with anorexia nervosa have a delusional belief that they are fat. Even though they are, in fact, actually emaciated. At the same time, those with bulimia nervosa fear becoming fat or getting fatter.

Anorexia nervosa is now recognized as a mental disorder; as a matter of fact, it is the mental disorder with the highest mortality. The illness remains controversial, but it is not uncommonly associated with other recognized mental diseases such as depression. Little is known about the factors that pave the way for the anorexic problem. However, various theories exist that are widely disputed. Patients can deteriorate until they are on the brink of death. And as a result, they often influence their family and others in a deleterious way.

Bulimia nervosa, in which subjects repeatedly induce postprandial vomiting, is associated with anorexia in some cases. The patient develops a distorted body image when they think they are fat, though in reality they are marasmic. They restrict and avoid food intake, though the bulimics may binge eat and then induce vomiting. Not all bulimics are underweight; some are slightly overweight, but they still suffer from physical and mental damage. The subject may become secretive, evasive, and dishonest, frequently hiding and destroying food as they are desperate to avoid gaining weight.

Someone may have told them that they look fat, or they themselves feel that they are obese. Sometimes, it may reflect their mother being fat. There is an association in some with sexual abuse at an early age, but this is not common. The patient's social life becomes nonexistent, particularly because there is animosity around any type of food. And they feel that they do not look good, so they become increasingly isolated. They rarely seek advice, though friends and relatives frequently call their attention to their alarming situation.

The fear of being fat, however, overwhelms any tendency to be honest or integral. Moreover, the compulsions the disease creates can continue and progress for many years. Treatment frequently fails, and multiple body organs can ultimately be damaged, sometimes permanently. Muscle wasting and weakness lead to profound fatigue and difficulty in performing day-to-day functions.

Orthostatic hypotension—which produces a feeling of weakness and unsteadiness with instability on standing, from the sitting position—is common and precipitated by an underlying low blood pressure and poor venous return to the heart.

Calcium deficiency leads to osteomalacia and osteoporosis, thinning and weakening of the bone, which predisposes to fractures following minor trauma. Hormonal imbalance is common, leading to irregularities in the menstrual cycle. Also, painful bone and joint disease is frequently witnessed, such as coccydynia, severe pain at the lower end of the spine, particularly experienced on sitting down. A common manifestation is the development of lanugo, the presence of soft, fine down or white hair on the face, back, and forearms. This is thought to be a response to hypersensitivity to cold and may be protective.

Mood swings and depression are common, often influenced by dehydration and electrolyte disturbance, hormone and vitamin deficiencies, and anorexia. This, in turn, is frequently associated with symptoms of obsessive-compulsive disorder. There may be a family history of depression.

Intellectual disturbances can also occur. However, often, the subjects of anorexia are highly intelligent, though introspective. The disease can have wide impacts, causing family problems and issues in the workplace. And they can be damaged by bullying when bullies detect their bodily damage and their subsequent weakness.

Prolonged fasting may damage the liver and is a major cause of liver failure in young people, and chronic heart failure, which could also produce adverse effects on the liver. Alcohol intake or abuse is rare in those who are anorexic.

Lowered body temperature and malnutrition can cause heart arrhythmias and heart failure, and vitamin and mineral deficiencies; vitamins A and C, iron, and iodine deficiencies can also occur. And they are associated with respiratory infections, kidney failure, visual disturbance, loss of teeth, and ultimately death.

Moreover, electrolyte disturbances can cause cardiac arrhythmias and even cardiac arrest. Low potassium levels can arrest the heart, causing cardiac muscle damage or even cardiac arrest. This causes the blood pressure to fall, resulting in orthostatic hypotension and a slow heart rate.

Neuromuscular disorders can occur as a result of vitamin and mineral deficiencies. Iron deficiency anemia frequently develops, impairing oxygen carriage to the tissues and causing breathlessness, weakness, infections, and heart arrhythmias.

Kidney failure is exacerbated by a combination of hypotension, electrolyte disturbances, protein deficiency, and urinary tract infections. Edema can result from low protein concentrations in the blood and the use of laxatives and diuretics.

Esophageal reflux is common, particularly in bulimia. And this can easily lead to damage in the lining of the esophagus and produce Barrett's esophagus, which can result in esophageal cancer. Vomiting in bulimia can cause a tear in the lining of the lower esophagus, the so-called "Mallory-Weiss syndrome." The fingers can become calloused by repeated vomiting, where the sufferer continuously shoves their fingers down the throat to induce vomiting. Vomiting can also damage tooth enamel, and dental problems are frequent, even sometimes resulting from scurvy.

Enhanced understanding in this area could prove to be a vital step in disrupting the dominant cultural constrictions underlying eating disorders. When health and management of illnesses are considered as personal moral responsibilities, people with body forms coded as different or abnormal have increasingly become the objects of media exposure. This can be damaging, particularly as the nature of the underlying disorders is not fundamentally understood.

Individuals with eating disorders resist the clinical labels that identify them. This can make the anorexic uncooperative or even hostile, thus exacerbating the problem. The media present slim, attractive women who are successful as a state to be strived for. Plus, the process of weight loss in achieving this may lead to anorexia. This will then accelerate and grow beyond the goal, leading to a distorted view of their own body image and an immense fear of reverting to an overweight state.

The patient who is severely affected by anorexia requires hospitalization and a cure for their malnutrition. This requires isolation, frequently intravenous nutrition, and in extreme situations, disconnection of washbasins in the room so that vomiting can be detected.

Following discharge from the hospital, the likelihood of relapse is very common. And ultimately, the only possibility of reversing the inexorable damage is dependent upon the patient voluntarily reversing the situation. And most people can get back to a normal lifestyle and maintain a normal healthy weight.

Binge eating disorders occur when a much larger amount of food than normal is taken in a short time. Bingeing can be a factor in bulimia, but it also occurs intermittently. What sets binge eating disorder apart from the other two disorders discussed above is the lack of purging and the high frequency of binge eating: two or more times weekly.

The triggers to binge eating are extremely mood sensitive, susceptible to hormonal changes, fatigue, life events, or disappointments with oneself or with others. Vulnerable sufferers may feel a binge coming on and gather food in advance or may just eat whatever is at hand, even food they don't ordinarily like.

Bingers usually eat alone, at home, in order to hide the amount or the types of food consumed. However, they also begin at a party or restaurant when a normal amount is eaten. But the overeating continues when they return home. The main issue is that once started, the binger feels out of control, compelled to keep eating to the point of discomfort and even misery. Subsequently, the binger feels ashamed and disgusted, but is unable to stop again and again. This leads to a chronic feeling of guilt and dread of discovery, thus addictive behavior.

Food cravings have a continuously disruptive effect on diet and ultimately goad us to binge eating behavior. Researchers have been teasing out the difference between craving, needing, and liking certain foods, irrespective of hunger. Virtually 100% of young women and 70% of young men have experienced food cravings during the past year.

Contrary to popular opinion, a craving is not in response to a body deficit of nutrients or calories. Food cravings, alcohol, and drug cravings all use the same brain pathways. The image of food or drugs invokes more intense reactions than the substance itself. This suggests the powerful role of habit, which is, in fact, reinforcing these biologically bound food cravings. The same pattern of increased craving is clearly demonstrated when a person attempts to stop smoking, another area where habits and cravings strongly develop.

Even after stopping, the former smoker may experience cravings when presented with any smoking-related situation or memory. So, too, certain life situations may bring on a food craving. Antidepressants and mood stabilizing medications might be useful in aiding mood regulation and dealing with craving and compulsive eating.

Once viewed as disorders of choice alone, eating disorders have been shown to have polygenetic factors in common with each other, as well as sharing risk factors with many psychiatric illnesses. Anorexia nervosa is the deadliest of all psychiatric disorders. Family and twin studies suggest that eating disorders run in families and are due to addictive genetic influences that affect food intake and body weight. Neuropeptides within the brain interact with gut-related peptides in a complex pattern, influencing appetite, the after-meal satiety point, and long-term body weight homeostasis.

Genetically susceptible obese patients may not respond normally to biological signals. Neuro-imaging studies are now being used to study brain reaction patterns to pictures, smells, tastes, and ideas in obese and normal weight persons.

One such project by nutritional researchers studied the PET scans of matched groups of obese and normal-weight men after consuming a tasty snack following a fast. The obese men had significantly greater regional blood flow in the emotional and impulsive areas of the brain than the normal weight men. This raises the question of whether obese patients have a qualitatively different taste response and decision-making pathway: a brain reward system, particularly sensitive to food, which reinforces their eating patterns by intensifying their brain reward responses.

Worldwide twin studies showed that the heritability of bulimia nervosa is between 50% and 83%. Environmental factors are less important, and the liability for developing bulimia nervosa is predominantly dependent on genetic factors. The remainder of the risk of developing bulimia nervosa comes from unique environmental factors or special stressors one may encounter. Anorexia nervosa also has genetic components, where heritability has been assessed as high as 60%. Anorexia nervosa and bulimia nervosa share related personality phenotypes such as perfectionism, body distraction, a drive for thinness, and obsessive-compulsive disorder.

BINGE EATING DISORDER

Bingeing is eating a much larger amount of food than normal in a short time, usually less than two hours. Bingeing is a factor common to nearly all of the eating disorders. What sets binge eating disorder apart from others is the lack of purging and the high frequency of bingeing, two or more times weekly.

In a prospective study of craving, participants were given a vanilla nutrition supplement drink as their total food for five days. If the participants lost weight, they were dropped from the study. The ratio of food cravings before the study was compared with food cravings during the study and during recovery. When participants could eat whatever they wanted, a normal control group ate as usual and were also given frequent samples of the vanilla drink. On the monotonous diet, food cravings peaked on the second day in all subjects.

Under MRI brain scans, subjects were asked to imagine their favorite food for 30 seconds, then take the vanilla nutrition drink for 30 seconds. Every participant showed MRI patterns of cravings while imagining their favorite food. The monopolist diet group had significantly more cravings than the normal diet group. This showed up in three craving-specific areas in the brain: the hippocampus, the insula, and the caudate nucleus. The same brain pathways may also be involved in feeding, not just in craving.

As mentioned earlier, food cravings, alcohol, and drug cravings all use the same brain pathways. The image of food or drugs invokes more intense reactions than the substance itself. This suggests the powerful role of habit in reinforcing these biologically bound food cravings. The same pattern of increased craving is clearly demonstrated when a person attempts to stop smoking, another area where habits and cravings strongly overlap.

Even after stopping, the former smoker may experience cravings when presented with any smoking-related situation or memory; also, certain life situations may bring on a food craving in those who are thus disposed.

BINGE EATING AND OTHER PSYCHIATRIC DISORDERS

Obese people with binge eating disorders have higher lifetime episodes of depression, panic disorder, generalized anxiety disorders, and bulimia than subjects without binge eating disorder. Those with binge eating behavior also show significantly higher rates of major depression, post-traumatic stress disorder, phobias, and alcohol dependency than non-bingers. Not surprisingly, this population has higher rates of medical comorbidities than non-bingers.

Other psychiatric conditions are also characterized in part by binge eating or increased eating. Bulimia is common in major depressive disorders and atypical depressions. In typical depression, a person eats too much and sleeps too much.

Women are far more likely to have this form of depression than men. Most depressed men actually lose weight during a depressive episode. Those with schizophrenia, schizoaffective disorder, and bipolar disorder have high rates of overweight and obesity.

In bipolar disorder, patients suffer from obesity almost twice as much as in the general population. Antipsychotic and other medications may compound the problem for these individuals by exacerbating eating and weight gain over long periods of time. Those with intellectual disabilities also tend to have elevated rates of overweight and obesity. They may not be able to regulate their own caloric intake for personal or environmental reasons.

In females, major depression during childhood is associated with obesity. The longer the depression, the more obese the adults become. Childhood abuse—sexual, physical, and verbal—also leads to an increased tendency toward overweight and obesity in adulthood, particularly in women. Childhood abuse can permanently alter a person's brain and adrenal gland reactions to stressful situations, which can lead to impaired eating.

PSYCHIATRIC TREATMENT OF MAJOR EATING DISORDERS

Obesity has just recently been declared to be a medical disorder in its own right. It is quite surprising because it is one of the most common and potentially fatal diseases of the present day. Treatment options for the psychiatric manifestations of obesity encompass medication and various types of psychotherapy.

All plans are based on a proper diet and an exercise program. As this overview shows, the wide range of social and genetic variables in each person who seeks treatment will necessitate specific treatments and a long-term commitment to weight normalization using all appropriate means of treatment.

To be successful, all psychotherapy must address emotional dysregulation, impulsive behavior, and cognitive/perceptual distortions. The latter includes body image and self-esteem issues as well as anxieties, which actually cause impulsive eating. Group and individual therapy—particularly cognitive behavioral therapy—can highlight rationalizations, reframe negative patterns of thinking, and also provide a more realistic manner of self-assessment. A recognition of one's own mental functioning and how one solves problems is crucial to change.

Anti-depressant drugs and mood stabilizing medications are useful in aiding mood regulation and dealing with craving and compulsive eating. Appetite suppressants need to be used long-term as well. Surgical treatment must have extensive medical follow-up and psychiatric and nutritional support. This calls for a high level of commitment by the patient to a permanent life change. One that involves a realistic timetable and a clear set of expectations and personal responsibilities that work out with the treatment team in the long run.

Understanding obesity as a medical disorder is seeing it as a dynamic pathological body state, arising from a convergence of genetic susceptibilities, and sustained by sociocultural and environmental influences on eating habits. Widely held prejudices against obese people as being lazy or morally weak should be confronted by all parties and dealt with openly. This must be done in order to change medical as well as social attitudes to the disorder. Public funding of preventive measures could begin a campaign of national awareness to stem this serious epidemic and its many complications and consequences, on a personal and national level.

DIET AND DEPRESSION

There is a considerable association between diet and mental health, both positive and negative. Low-calorie diets, below 1200 calories, promote depression. A recent study shows that even short-term caloric restriction—which usually fails—can be associated with mental disorders.

Yo-yo dieting usually ends in overall weight gain. Commercial forces determine the nature of food intake. This is also affected immensely by government policy. Governments need to look at the food industry, as the responsibility is not entirely individual. Ultra-processed foods obtained in the supermarket undoubtedly promote weight gain.

CHAPTER 10: PHYSICAL ACTIVITY AND BODY WEIGHT

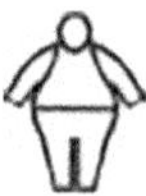

The importance of energy expenditure has already been stressed; it remains a fundamental issue involving weight stability. Physical inactivity is a major factor in the present-day weight dilemma that afflicts so many American citizens.

Individuals vary widely in terms of their energy expenditure as a result of their differing physical activity. While a number of people run marathons, far more individuals refrain from indulging in any form of physical activity at all. Physical energy expenditure ranges from static physical exercise, such as rapidly increasing and decreasing muscle tone, gesticulating, to voluntarily moving in athletic activity, as in running.

EXERCISE

- Exercise is good.
- Weight training is better!
- Select a regimen you can easily comply with.
- Don't overdo it in the beginning.
- Walking is excellent!

The energy expenditure of minimal daily activity in a non-exercising person is about 50% greater than the basal metabolic rate. The latter is the amount of expenditure required to maintain the stability of the individual while totally resting, such as lying in bed. Moderately active individuals add approximately another 20% to this figure.

Obesity in itself, once established, limits physical activity and prohibits most forms of athletics. Females tend to expend fewer calories through physical activity than do males. It has also been suggested that obese individuals are likely to show a limited variety of fine movements: moving around in the chair and gesticulating, rather than those who are of normal weight.

ENERGY EXPENDITURE AND EXERCISE

- **Day-to-day normal activities:** 500 to 1000 cal
- **Walking:** 300 cal per hour
- **Cycling:** 400 cal per hour
- **Running:** 500 to 600 cal per hour
- **Rowing:** 600 cal per hour
- **Swimming:** 400 to 600 cal per hour

Studies comparing the body composition in heavy and light workers show that these groups have similar fat content. Clearly, those engaged in light work should modify their food intake to maintain the same sort of equilibrium as the heavy worker. The overall effects of physical exercise in relation to total energy turnover each day are relatively small.

However, it has been shown that those who walk more weigh less. Furthermore, the decline in physical activity in the population as a whole probably contributes to the increased prevalence of obesity. The exact mechanism is not fully understood. Whatever the cause of obesity, it can be argued that increased physical activity is a useful aid to weight reduction and to maintaining reduced body weight. However, it is not as simple as just burning up more calories by, for example, running.

EXERCISE PROGRAMS

It is usually necessary to walk in excess of 30 minutes a day to establish any significant weight loss. Unfortunately, for those beginning a heavy exercise program involving 30 minutes of exercise daily, fewer than 30% will persist for any significant length of time to make a substantial impact. Most studies emphasizing exercise programs have shown a very high attrition rate, even when these trials last only a few weeks or months. More intense forms of exercise than walking, such as jogging, are more likely to result in a lack of long-term compliance.

Losing weight by exercise, therefore, depends considerably upon the motivation of the individual. The increase in work output was seen to affect total energy turnover to only a small extent. We all see thousands of people indulging in marathons such as the "London Marathon." Running a marathon only burns up something along the lines of 3500 calories; this amount can easily be eaten in a day.

It is possible that the decrease in activity that occurs with age may form the basis for the decline in muscle mass and lean body mass as people grow older. Replacement of lean tissue by fat associated with aging worsens the problem of energy imbalance since the basal need for energy falls with the total reduction in metabolically active lean tissue. This ultimately leads to a further drop in the basal metabolic rate and the tendency to gain body fat.

Everyone entering weight reduction programs should be aware that the physiological beneficial effects of short periods of moderately intense exercise are well-documented. And the fact that a minimum of 20 minutes of moderate activity added at least three times a week is good for the cardiovascular system. This kind of activity also seems to play an important role in improving an individual's sense of well-being, probably by the production of endorphins. It is unclear whether this amount of exercise helps to maintain lean body mass. Not only are the effects of aerobic exercise positive, but working with weights increases the ratio of body protein to body fat. This is beneficial and also stimulates metabolic activity. Exercise is also good for the brain!

"Walking 4,000 steps per day, just less than 2 miles for most, could be enough to reduce the risk of early death," researchers say. Health experts had previously called people "sedentary" if they managed fewer than 5,000 steps. And to be fair, the recent craze for recording your daily total, with items such as Fitbits, has led to a target of 10,000 steps per day being recommended. An analysis of 227,000 healthy people from 17 studies found that the possibility of dying prematurely can be cut by thirty percent in people who walk 4,000 steps a day.

This study found that the chances of dying from cardiovascular disease, heart attacks, and strokes start to lessen if they walk 2500 steps daily. It was emphasized that the more steps taken, the better, with every extra thousand steps being linked to a 15% reduction in someone's risk of dying prematurely. (This review was published in the European Journal of Preventive Cardiology in 2023.)

CHAPTER 11: NUTRITIONAL FACTS AND FIGURES

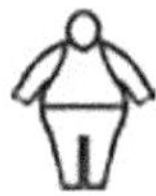

Depending upon size, age, and activity level, an adult woman typically needs an intake of about 1700 to 2000 calories per day; the typical adult male needs 2000 to 2500 calories. With increasing age, calorific requirements fall.

To lose one pound of fat in a week, a person needs to reduce their overall calorie intake by 3500 calories, or the approximate equivalent of two days of food; it's tough! To lose fat, one should not concentrate on eating less fat per se. It is the total caloric intake that adds weight, and easily taken carbohydrates produce as much weight gain in pounds of fat per calorie as does fat itself. It is not just a question of eating fewer calories, though. An adequate diet must comprise essential vitamins and minerals, irrespective of the fact that these can be covered by over-the-counter medications available in pharmacies and health stores.

CHOLESTEROL

Cholesterol is a waxy lipid that is an essential constituent of every cell in the body. It is manufactured in the liver as well as being ingested. Lipoproteins carry cholesterol from the liver through the body via the bloodstream. As mentioned earlier, bad cholesterol is low-density lipoprotein (LDL). This contributes to cardiac and vascular disease.

High-density lipoprotein (HDL) "sweeps up" some of the cholesterol deposits and is therefore regarded as good cholesterol. High levels of LDL-cholesterol lead to heart disease. But avoiding foods that are high in cholesterol does not necessarily decrease the amount of cholesterol in the blood.

Saturated fats used to be considered the main culprit for vascular disease: fats that are present in dairy products raise high-density lipoproteins as well as low-density lipoproteins, so that a balance is maintained.

Another type of fat, trans fats, is partially hydrogenated vegetable oil. This oil increases LDL cholesterol and decreases HDL cholesterol. This causes the depositing of cholesterol on blood vessels without the mopping-up factor of HDL cholesterol being present. Trans fats are present in large amounts in fried foods, chips, cookies, and cakes. These substances, in themselves, contain no cholesterol. However, they stimulate cholesterol production by the liver.

REFINED CARBOHYDRATES

Fat, however, is not the real enemy. Eating fat does not make you fat; conversely, it can help you to eat less overall. Refined carbohydrates—which cause the blood sugar to shoot up rapidly—are the main enemy. Not all carbohydrates are bad!

Many vegetables and fruits are high in vitamins and minerals. They also contain antioxidants that dispose of potentially harmful oxygen byproducts called free radicals. These substances also contain fiber. Fiber can lower cholesterol and stabilize blood sugar levels.

In giving dietary advice, therefore, one should recommend a strategy of eating in moderation and avoiding trans fats and refined carbohydrates. Instead, eat foods that are minimally processed, such as brown rice, blueberries, and fish sautéed with garlic and olive oil.

MEAT

In preparing meat, external fats should be removed. Portions should be restricted to the size of the palm of the hand. Expensive cuts of beef taste better as they contain more fat! Veal is low in fat but high in cholesterol. Lamb and pork tend to contain a lot of fat. Cutting the fat from pork leaves healthy lean meat. Bacon is high in sodium and fat, and sausages are high in carbohydrates and fat.

FISH

Fish—particularly salmon, mackerel, and sardines—are an excellent source of omega-3 fatty acids. They are rich in calcium. Farm-raised salmon and tuna may accumulate high levels of mercury and other toxins, such as minute particles of plastic. It is safer to eat wild salmon rather than the now ubiquitous farm-raised salmon, which again is more expensive. Batter-dipped white fish are high in fat, particularly the trans fats. Shellfish are high in cholesterol but low in calories; their cholesterol is not usually significant enough to boost levels in the bloodstream.

CHICKEN

High in protein, low in fat and cholesterol, chicken, without skin, makes for healthy eating. Turkey is the leanest meat of all. And with the skin removed, the fat content of turkey breast is less than 1%. Duck, from which the skin is removed, is contrary to popular belief, low in fat! Game birds, such as pheasant, are very low in fat.

Wild game, like deer, is a good source of protein and is also low in fat.

DAIRY PRODUCTS

Milk contains calcium, protein, zinc, and fat-soluble vitamins. Cheese is similar to milk. Eggs are high in cholesterol, though the whites are an excellent source of protein, and the yolks are not necessarily bad. Yogurt is good, but tends to be sweetened with refined sugar.

All the while, bacon, eggs, and sausage fried in butter are not a healthy combination of foodstuffs. Margarines—which are free of trans fat and contain twice as much polyunsaturated as saturated fat—are a healthy source of fat. Vegetable oils are excellent. They contain large amounts of heart-healthy omega-3 and omega-6 fatty acids.

OTHER FOODS

Nuts contain a large amount of fat but also many beneficial nutrients, such as the B vitamins. They are good in small amounts. Coconuts are high in phytosterols: compounds that have been shown to reduce levels of blood cholesterol. They are, however, also high in saturated fat and carbohydrates but contain no cholesterol.

Vital nutrients are plentiful in seeds, which also contain fiber and frequently omega-3 fatty acids. Flax seeds are particularly high in omega-3 fatty acids and have anticoagulant properties. They may also be useful in treating some tumors.

Soy protein is the only complete vegetable protein that contains all of the essential amino acids. Soy also contains iron, calcium, magnesium, vitamin D, riboflavin, thiamine, folate, and good fats. Soy flour is higher in protein and lower in carbohydrate than wheat flour, and it lacks gluten. Legumes are low in fat and contain no cholesterol. They are rich in minerals and fiber. Hummus contains a high concentration of fat.

CEREALS

Bread is high in calories and carbohydrates. Croissants are the most calorie-dense. A bagel can contain 400 calories. Whole wheat bread is the lowest in calories and highest in fiber. Muffins need not be so calorie-dense, but they contain trans fatty acids. Pasta is low in fat and cholesterol, although high in carbohydrates.

Moreover, rice is rich in carbohydrates, low in fat and cholesterol, and a good source of B vitamins. Whole grains digest slowly. And therefore, they don't produce rapid rises in blood glucose levels. Most cereals are a rich source of carbohydrates; other nutrients may be added. Of all the cereal grains and grasses, oats are the most nutritious. They provide more protein than rice, and they contain B vitamins, iron, selenium, and fiber.

FRUITS AND VEGETABLES

Fruits and vegetables are important to a healthy diet. They are rich in antioxidants and contain vitamins, minerals, and fiber. The highest in antioxidants are blueberries. At the same time, blue, red, and purple berries are high in anthocyanins. The healthiest of all the vegetables is *asparagus*. Carrots are rich in vitamin A. Onions and garlic have mild anticoagulant properties and are effective in preventing thrombosis in vessels.

FAST FOODS

Probably the biggest contemporary problem that afflicts us in relation to obesity is the social trend, or compulsion, to eat in fast food restaurants or takeaways. A single meal of a super burger, jumbo fries, mega soda, and fried pie greatly increases the daily recommended caloric requirements and is high in sodium yet alarmingly deficient in vitamins and minerals. Just the beef part of a double burger contains 560 calories with 33g of fat and 47g of carbohydrate. Whether purchased from McDonald's or Burger King, the calorific counts are similar.

Kentucky Fried Chicken contains a large amount of fat in the batter and in the skin. An Extra Crispy Breast contains 470 calories, and a "Chunky Chicken Pot Pie" exudes 770 calories. Taco Bell's products tend to be lower in cholesterol. However, taco salad with a shell (crust) contains a staggering 800 calories! This makes the taco salad higher in calories, saturated fat, carbohydrates, and sodium than a "Big Mac" or a "Whopper." It is the crust that causes the problem.

The health message, as far as pizza is concerned, is "go for the finest crust, least cheese, and most vegetables." One slice of "Beef Personal Plan" at Pizza Hut contains 710 calories. Veggie pizzas on the thin crust are probably best. But pizzas do not promote healthy eating and are best avoided.

CHAPTER 12: NUTRITION AND METABOLISM

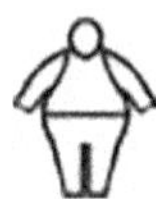

Under resting conditions, a normal healthy adult male burns approximately 10 calories per pound of body weight per day. With normal activity, this caloric requirement virtually doubles. The caloric requirement is met by the use of the three main foodstuffs, carbohydrates, fats, and proteins. The body initially burns the carbohydrates, glucose, and glycogen, but it stores and contains small quantities of each.

And therefore, fasting will lead to fat and protein being burned. The basic requirement of living cells is to use protein for the repair and replacement of cells and to supply the energy to drive these reactions. In order to fuel the required metabolic activities, the body needs to generate a substance, adenosine triphosphate (ATP).

CARBOHYDRATE METABOLISM

The gut rapidly breaks down complex sugars into simple ones, predominantly glucose, fructose, and galactose. Sugars are absorbed through the small intestine and transported to the liver. Some of the glucose remains in the circulation to maintain the blood sugar at a constant level. It is transported to cells to provide energy. Glucose is broken down in the cells by a process known as glycolysis, which requires oxygen.

FAT METABOLISM

About 40% of calories in the average American diet are derived from fat. Fats and oils are triesters of glycerol and various fatty acids. The ability of lipids to be stored in the body as fat provides the source for continuous energy production. Fats are used once carbohydrate stores have been metabolized, which is usually after a period of about 12 hours of starvation.

Absorption of lipids depends upon their being mixed with bile, and then they are absorbed in the small intestine and converted into triglycerides. They are then transported via the lymphatic system or directly into the bloodstream. Fat is not only stored but is also used to form a key component of cell membranes. A reduction in carbohydrate intake causes an increase in the breakdown of triglycerides and free fatty acids.

Virtually all tissues, except the brain, require lipids as an energy source. When excessive amounts of lipids are metabolized and used for energy, breakdown products (which accumulate in the bloodstream), such as acetoacetic acid, give rise to a condition known as ketosis. Criticism of the Atkins diet is that it has led to the production of ketosis.

PROTEIN METABOLISM

The main function of protein is to provide the building blocks for cells. Proteins can be utilized as a fuel source for energy in times of stress. Protein molecules taken in the diet are broken down by digestion into peptides and amino acids. These are the basic constituents of all larger protein molecules. There is a high turnover of body protein. And many grams of protein are carried throughout the body per hour. The integral components of protein, amino acids, are linked to cellular proteins and stored as protein.

Once the cell is replete, unused excess and amino acids are converted to keto acids. A breakdown product of amino acids is ammonia. This, in large amounts, is toxic and depresses brain function. Protein is imperative for the production of the nucleic acids, DNA and RNA. They are also instrumental to the core genetic structure of man.

NUTRITIONAL REQUIREMENTS

Nutritional requirements vary with age, sex, and body size. And they can be influenced by drugs, hormones, and disease states. Carbohydrates provide approximately half of the human energy requirement. They may be ingested as simple sugars or more complex carbohydrates. Certain tissues—such as the brain, blood cells, and the kidneys—have an obligatory requirement for glucose.

Lipids, as well as being a source of energy, play an important role in the structure and function of cells. Proteins, unlike carbohydrates and lipids, are not held in storage. They do, however, make up approximately 20% of the lean body mass as muscle.

Proteins exist in the form of enzymes, which are required to enable chemical reactions to be carried out inside the body. Another important role of proteins is to provide a source of essential amino acids. These are the acids that are needed for normal body function but cannot be produced spontaneously by the body. Dietary proteins contain these essential amino acids in varying concentrations.

Many of the normal chemical processes essential for life require vitamins. Deficiencies in these vitamins result in well-defined diseases. A total of 13 vitamins have been identified as being essential in normal human nutrition.

Five of these are fat-soluble and eight are water-soluble. Fat-soluble vitamins are A, D, E, and K. Vitamins A, C, and E, together with the mineral selenium, are antioxidants crucial for the breakdown of free radical oxidation products, which are damaging.

Deficiencies of individual vitamins produce well-known syndromes. One of the best-known diseases to the public is “scurvy,” which historically was common on long sea voyages. Scurvy, which occurs through bleeding from the gums, is due to a deficiency in vitamin C or ascorbic acid.

On long transatlantic sea voyages, sailors became deficient in vitamin C and developed a full-blown syndrome of scurvy, which ultimately became treatable by the provision of limes to sailors embarking on such long voyages, hence the term limeys for British sailors.

In addition to vitamins, there are 19 minerals and trace minerals that are essential to humans. And they may be grouped into four categories based on their function. Calcium, phosphorus, magnesium, and zinc are structural components of bone. A second group, sodium, potassium, and chloride, operates as major charged ions within the cellular mechanism.

Calcium and magnesium are both structural components of bone and function as charged ions. Trace minerals, which are necessary for normal health, include iron, zinc, copper, selenium, manganese, molybdenum, cobalt, iodine, and chromium.

Minerals are essential to prevent deficiency states. And the intake of minerals can be low even in the obese, but particularly so following surgery for morbid obesity. Malabsorption—the consequence of a number of diseases and the effects of some drugs—can alter mineral balances.

Calcium is the most abundant mineral in the body and plays a vital role in muscular and cardiac activity. It is also involved in the coagulation of the blood and the secretion of certain hormones. Excessive intakes of vitamins A and D can give rise to high levels of calcium.

Low levels of calcium may be associated with low levels of albumin and magnesium. Magnesium is an important mineral within cells and is involved in many chemical reactions. Levels of magnesium frequently fall following obesity surgery. Conversely, too much can cause cell damage and renal failure.

Trace elements also tend to be depleted after obesity surgery. A common manifestation of zinc deficiency is hair loss; this may go along with a deficiency of the B group of vitamins, such as biotin. The body usually responds promptly to the replacement of the missing zinc and biotin. Iron levels may also suffer, and in association with this, anemia may develop.

ASSESSMENT OF THE NUTRITIONAL STATE

The body mass index—sometimes referred to as Quetelet's index—when of the order of 20 to 25, is associated with a good general standard of health. Once the obese range is entered, mortality increases markedly with increasing weight. Numerous methods have been developed to estimate the amount of fatty tissue in the human body. Among the simplest is the anthropometric technique of skinfold thickness. In fact, the triceps skinfold is most commonly used.

Here, the skin and underlying tissues superficial to the triceps muscle group at the back of the upper arm are pinched together, and the thickness of the skinfold is measured. The fat thickness is also measured over other muscles in the body, in particular over the shoulders, abdomen, and thighs. The skin fold thicknesses are compared with those expressed in tables for differing degrees of obesity.

Skeletal muscle can be estimated by using another anthropometric technique, that of mid-arm circumference.

This is the measurement of lean arm tissue, which is then compared with existing standards. The mid-arm circumference is calculated by subtracting the mid-arm fat circumference from the mid-arm total circumference using a mathematical formula.

More sophisticated methods of measuring body fat include *densitometry*. This involves the patient being submerged in water, and imaging techniques such as computerized tomography and ultrasound. Electrical conductivity or impedance measurements can also be used to estimate body fat. They are, in turn, based on the difference in conductivity of lean and fat tissue.

CHAPTER 13: CONSERVATIVE METHODS OF TREATING OBESITY

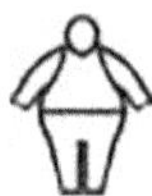

The task of losing a large amount of weight and sustaining the reduction is always major. To lose 100 pounds which many people need to do, if you try to achieve a negative balance of input over output of energy of 1000 cal per day it would take you 13 months and achieving a 1000 cal per day negative balance is not easy, it requires a strict adherence to a dietary regimen with supplemental exercise and modification of lifestyle. If a person is 100 pounds overweight, he or she is carrying 100 pounds of excess fat. And this roughly amounts to 400,000 calories that they need to lose.

OVER-THE-COUNTER DIETS

A wide variety of methods are in use for unsupervised slimming. Many magazines are devoted to the subject. And, normally, supermarkets display the slimmest breads and crisps as well as low-energy soft drinks. Over-the-counter items—like meat loaf-based products—are deemed to reduce hunger by providing bulk to fill the stomach. They are also widely available. However, there is no scientific evidence that these are of any value in reducing food intake or producing weight loss in the long term. Furthermore, some vegetarian diet dishes bought in supermarkets could comprise a lot of calories due to additives containing carbohydrates and fats.

UNSUPERVISED DIETARY ADVICE

- Magazines
- Newspapers
- Television
- Internet
- Random crash diets

Calorie-counted meals are widely available in supermarkets, and the recordings of the calorific value of foods in restaurants are becoming more popular, but there is no evidence that they can be relied upon as a vehicle for long-term weight loss.

Organizations and magazines run self-help groups. The magazines give substantive advice on slimming, but often perpetrate incorrect nutritional principles. They frequently advocate crash diets. These diets tend to almost invariably lead to a rebound weight gain. Or, in other instances, they focus on specific foodstuffs that may be inappropriate for a long-term strategy in achieving weight loss. The most successful of the self-help organizations is "Weight Watchers (WW)," which we will discuss in more detail.

Historically, diets have focused on reduced fat intake. For over half a century, emphasis has been placed by the medical profession on lowering cholesterol and reducing the intake of animal fat in dairy products. Now, the focus has shifted to reducing carbohydrate intake. And carbohydrate excesses are converted into fat and are the major problem underlying the obese state today. You should let the right foods be your meds!

Eat more green plants, broccoli, cauliflower, asparagus, zucchini, berries, particularly blueberries, and nuts, and avoid processed foods. A study in 2019 of 20,000 men and women aged between 21 and 90 years found that a diet high in processed foods resulted in an 18% increased risk of death due to these major killers.

Successful slimming is difficult and clearly depends on a number of factors. Many factors are not appreciated subjectively, but the subject's ability to keep to a particular dietary regimen is as important as total energy intake. Most individuals find it difficult to sustain any regimen for a prolonged period of time. This is necessary! Yet still, some diets may be complicated, hard to produce, and expensive.

DIETS

- Over-the-counter
- Methyl cellulose—swells in the stomach, of no value
- Calorie-free diet soda—useful
- Magazines and diet books—on the whole, of no proven value

NAMED DIETS

- Low-fat—Ornish (fat is nine calories per gram)
- Low carbohydrate—Atkins (carbohydrates are four calories per gram)
- Other low-carbohydrate diets—Sugar Busters, South Beach

CALORIE COUNTING DIETS

When taking calorie-counting diets, the subject is allowed to eat any foods that cumulatively stay within a given energy intake. Although there is freedom of choice, there are many disadvantages. Food needs to be weighed precisely as energy intake is calculated from this. But this can be difficult.

Commonly, patients will state that these diets fail. However, in reality, it is unlikely that the patient has managed to adhere strictly to the dietary requirements. A slight variation on this theme is the set diet, in which a diet sheet provides the week's menu for three meals per day. These menus offer variety, and alternatives are frequently given. They are diets such as "Nutrisystem," which provide a rich variety of food. However, these diets are in very small portions, and by no means have the healthiest food items. Some vegetarian diet meals bought in supermarkets, as stated, can be very high in calories.

Eating an additional 1% would mean an extra 10,000 calories per year. This is 1 1/4 cans of cola per day and will cause a gain of two pounds per year: the equivalent of walking 100 miles!

LOW-FAT DIETS

With low-fat diets, the individual is provided with a list of foods that are high in fat and must be avoided or severely restricted. These diets often originated specifically with the object of reducing cholesterol levels, thereby reducing the risk of heart disease. Carbohydrates are not usually restricted to these diets. As a result, they are prone to failure.

LOW CARBOHYDRATE DIETS

Diets that are low in carbohydrates are the key to weight reduction and have actually been available for many years. Dr. Frederick Banting—who discovered insulin over a century ago—devised low-carbohydrate diets for treating diabetes.

While they have been used over the years, emphasis has only recently been placed on them regarding weight loss. This is the case because it has now been realized that carbohydrates are the real enemy. The most widely used low-carbohydrate diets are the South Beach Diet, Sugar Busters, and the Atkins diet.

The South Beach Diet

The South Beach Diet claims to promote selective carbohydrates and allow low amounts of fat. The aim is to reach reliance on the right carbohydrates and the right fats: the good ones, and enable the patient to live quite happily without bad carbohydrates and bad fats. The claim is that between eight and 13 pounds in weight can be lost in the first two weeks. This is achieved by eating normal-sized helpings of chicken, turkey, fish, and shellfish.

Vegetables are encouraged in the diet, which also includes eggs and nuts. Salads are encouraged to use olive oil as a dressing, but avoid other high-calorie dressings such as mayonnaise. Three balanced meals a day are allowed, and eating until one's hunger is satisfied is encouraged. A dessert may be taken, but only after dinner.

Bread, rice, potatoes, pasta, and baked goods are completely prohibited. All the while, fruit is restricted in the early days of the diet. Cakes, cookies, ice cream, and sugar are also banned. Some alcohol is allowed. However, it should be restricted to 15 units per week for men and 12 units per week for women. It is claimed that most of the weight loss in the first few weeks comes off the abdomen. As a result, clothes sizes are influenced early.

Physical cravings for food usually disappear as long as the patient adheres to the program. It is claimed that patients wind up eating fewer food items that created these urges in the first place. And also, fewer foods that cause the body to store excess fat.

Allows lean:

- Beef
- Pork
- Veal
- Lamb

- Eggs
- Chicken
- Turkey
- Fish Nuts
- Low-fat cheeses
- Olive oil
- Canola oil

Encourages salads, eggs, cheese, nuts, and olive oil. Bans bread, rice, potatoes, pasta, cake, cereal, cookies, and ice cream.

After the first two weeks, phase 2 of the diet is entered. Here, fruit is allowed, along with a small amount of rice or cereal. The subject continues on this phase until the ideal weight is achieved, which may take several months. Thereafter, in phase 3, the subject is requested to permanently stay on a less restricted form of this phase of the diet. And this will eventually become a way of life in the long term.

It is important to note that the South Beach Diet was devised by Arthur Agatson, a cardiologist who became disillusioned with the low-fat, high carbohydrate diet that the American Heart Association recommended. As a consequence, he introduced the South Beach Diet in the mid-1990s.

Focus was still placed on the prevention of the myriad of heart and vascular problems that stem from the obese state. While paying attention to the beneficial effects on the cardiovascular system, Dr. Agatston also realizes the importance of the cosmetic effects of losing weight, as a strong motivating factor for continuation with the diet. The physiological lift that comes from an improved appearance benefits the entire person and keeps many patients from backsliding. The end result is cardiovascular health with better, more active, and more positive habitus and attitude. The diet is also aimed at treating the other major killers.

An important principle of the South Beach Diet is to permit good carbohydrates and vegetables. Ultimately, fruits and whole grains may be taken to curtail the bad carbohydrates: the highly processed ones from which all of the fiber has been stripped away during the manufacturing process.

To make up for the cut in carbohydrates, the diet permits the intake of fats and animal proteins. The reason for this is that the so-called heart-healthy diets were very difficult to adhere to as they relied too heavily on the dieter's ability to eat low-fat foods over the long term.

In a nutshell, the South Beach Diet encourages lean beef, pork, veal, and lamb, provided the fat is removed. This diet also permits eggs. Eggs contain a lot of vitamin D and have a positive effect on the balance between good and bad cholesterol. And hence, they can be taken. An egg only contains 60 to 70 calories and is good in moderation.

Chicken, turkey, fish, especially the oily ones like salmon, tuna, and mackerel, are recommended. In addition, nuts, low-fat cheeses, and yogurt are considered optimal. Olive oil, canola oil, and peanut oil are permitted in moderation as these items contain the good fats. This diet allows some carbohydrates because severe limitation can lead to a breakdown of fats, producing ketosis.

To otherwise healthy overweight individuals, this diet is not harmful. However, it may be associated with a decrease in blood volume and some dehydration. And this could, in the long term, possibly affect kidney function. It is therefore helpful to drink large volumes of fluid, up to eight glasses of water.

In a clinical trial including 40 overweight volunteers, the South Beach Diet was compared to the American Heart Association low-fat program. After 12 weeks, five patients in the American Heart Association diet had given up compared with just one on the South Beach plan.

South Beach dieters experienced a mean weight loss of 13.6 pounds, almost double the 7.5 pounds lost by the Heart Association group. Those on the South Beach Diet also showed a greater decrease in waist-to-hip ratio, thus suggesting a real decrease in cardiac risk and providing a positive psychological effect.

Cholesterol levels dramatically decreased for those on the South Beach Diet. Moreover, their good-to-bad cholesterol ratio improved more than that of those in the American Heart Association diet. In addition, much of the insulin resistance syndrome disappeared within the first few weeks on the South Beach Diet. The cravings for sugars and starches were also virtually gone.

After two weeks, fruits and bran or oatmeal are allowed. At this stage, a little whole grain bread can also be introduced into the diet. It should not be spread with jelly, but a light covering of butter is allowed. Potatoes are banned! Eggs should be boiled or poached and not fried. Fruits with the lowest glycemic index are strawberries, blueberries, and raspberries, and they are encouraged.

Meanwhile, bananas have a high glycemic index and should be avoided; tomato ketchup is not allowed. Tomato slices, however, are fine. Lettuce, pickles, and onions are perfect! Green peppers, garlic, mushrooms, mustard, and olives are good. Raw broccoli is excellent. Broccoli is covered with a layer of nutritious fiber, and the carbohydrate content is slowly absorbed.

Not only is the frying of potatoes bad, but even when boiled, the glycemic index remains high. Why? Because boiling makes the carbohydrate content more suitable for rapid absorption. The digestion of fats and proteins, along with carbohydrates—which is allowed—slows the speed with which the carbohydrates themselves are rendered suitable for absorption. And, therefore, prevents a rapid rise in blood sugar concentration.

A little olive oil will enhance the process of slowing down the absorption of carbohydrates, hence the practice, which is often recommended, of taking a spoonful of Metamucil. And a glass of water about 15 minutes before a meal.

Insoluble fiber mixed with the food has the effect of slowing the speed at which the stomach digests food. Also, the rate at which the stomach empties is slowed, thus reducing the rate of absorption of carbohydrates.

WORD OF WARNING: THE IMPORTANCE OF WHAT WE DRINK

In many ways, what we drink is more critical than what we eat! The stomach empties liquids more rapidly than solids, rendering them suitable for quick absorption. And, thus, carbohydrates containing liquids have an extremely high glycemic index, leading to a rapid increase in blood sugar concentrations.

As has been pointed out, there is something of the order of nine or 10 teaspoons of sugar in a can of Coke. If pure water is drunk, it has the effect of diluting the content of the stomach and slowing down the absorption of solid foods. Therefore, drinking as much water as you can is recommended.

Beer has a high glycemic index as a result of its maltose content. This makes it even worse than table sugar. Coffee may be protective to the heart and is, therefore, not discouraged; it can, however, stimulate the stomach to secrete more acid and thereby increase the rate of digestion. A further effect of this is that the increased rate of gastric emptying may increase appetite.

Tea also contains a large amount of caffeine. It may also be useful in the prevention of cardiac disease and possibly even prostate cancer. According to the protagonist of the South Beach Diet, wine is less damaging than white bread; it is less fattening.

AUGMENTING THE SOUTH BEACH DIET (ACCORDING TO CARDIOLOGIST DR. AGATSTON)

- Aspirin
- Multivitamin preparations
- Fish oil-omega-3 fatty acids
- Cholesterol-lowering drugs such as Lipitor or Zocor, if indicated. Possibly testosterone gel

THE GLYCEMIC INDEX OF FOOD

The amount that the food in question increases your blood sugar compared with the amount that the same weight of white bread would increase it. Avoid white bread as per the glycemic index of 100.

Glycemic indices that are greater than 100:

- Doughnuts
- Waffles
- Gluten-free bread
- French baguettes
- Bagels
- Watermelons
- Mashed potato
- French fries
- Baked potato, the highest, 158%
- Foods with glycemic indices less than 20:
- Artichoke
- Asparagus
- Broccoli

- Brussels sprouts
- Cabbage
- Cauliflower
- Celery
- Cucumbers
- Beets
- Kale
- Mustard greens
- Spinach
- Turnips
- Mushrooms
- Nuts (but these have a high fat content)
- Peas
- Green beans
- The glycemic index of sugars:
- Glucose: 137%
- Maltose: 150%
- Lactose: 92%
- Fructose: 32%
- The glycemic index in fruits:
- GOOD
- Strawberries
- Blueberries
- Raspberries
- Red or black berries
- BAD
- Bananas
- The glycemic index of alcohols:
- Best: red wine
- Cardiac benefits: whiskey
- Worst: beer (high maltose)

OUTCOMES ACHIEVED WITH THE SOUTH BEACH DIET

It is common for people to lose eight to 12 pounds during the first two weeks of the South Beach Diet. This is very encouraging for diet participants. Yet, most of the initial weight loss is due to the loss of carbohydrate intake. This results in a loss of water storage and loss from restricting carbohydrate intake, equalizing after about 10 to 14 days. Shortly thereafter, weight loss slows. A similar result can be achieved by suddenly stopping copious amounts of alcohol intake.

Proponents of the South Beach Diet strongly recommend an exercise program. But, in moderation, so that the exercise program becomes only a slight intervention in normal lifestyle rather than a major new all-consuming discipline.

For most people, a brisk 20-minute daily walk is recommended. However, it can only be expected to burn about 100 calories. The majority of the benefit from exercise is gained during the first 20 minutes. Weight training has many benefits. It improves muscle-to-fat ratio, increases metabolism, and enables the body to burn fuel faster, even when sleeping.

Increasing lean body mass, that is, body weight from anything other than fat, has a helpful effect on weightlifting. Weight training is also helpful for women in preventing osteoporosis. Furthermore, exercise lowers blood pressure and increases good cholesterol.

The developer of the South Beach Diet, Agaston, who is a cardiologist—in addition to adhering to his own diet to promote further weight loss—takes aspirin and fish oil capsules and uses testosterone gel. Body pump classes are a very good form of exercise: the burning of increased calories can continue for up to six hours after stopping the exercise.

The proponents of the South Beach Diet place great emphasis on eating patterns. Multiple meals stimulate less overall secretion of insulin than one or two large feedings. Large feedings are dangerous as they produce a peak of sugar absorption and insulin secretion. And they also manage to promote insulin resistance.

Long periods of fasting alter the body's response to insulin by causing it to enter the conservation mode. This causes fat storage. It is therefore recommended that people should strive to consume three balanced meals per day with an absence of snacking between them. And the longer the period between them, the more beneficial it will be to retain good health.

THE SUGAR BUSTERS DIET

The Sugar Busters diet emphasizes that sugar is toxic. It is stressed that overproduction of insulin causes the body to store excess sugar as fat, which creates insulin resistance. Insulin further inhibits the mobilization of previously stored fat. And then, insulin signals the liver to make cholesterol. As a result, too much sugar is clearly bad.

The Sugar Busters diet selectively prohibits carbohydrates that culminate in an intense insulin response. These are refined sugars. Foods that must be eliminated from the diet are potatoes, corn, white rice, bread from refined flour, beets, carrots, granulated sugar, corn syrup, molasses, honey, sugar, sweets, and beer.

Red wine is allowed in the Sugar Busters diet. For those who consume alcoholic beverages, the one that is most beneficial appears to be red wine. Populations in countries with a high relative consumption of red wine compared to other spirits experience a lower rate of cardiovascular disease. Alcohol, however, is high in calories. With the Sugar Busters diet, as with all diets, exercise is regarded as a definite plus.

THE STRATEGY OF THE SUGAR BUSTERS DIET

- To modulate insulin production by withdrawing sugars with a high glycemic index.
- Multiple small meals are preferable to one or two large ones.
- Calories are not counted.
- Drinking large amounts of water is encouraged.

Modulating insulin is, therefore, the key component of the Sugar Busters diet. Successfully controlling insulin allows the patient to unlock improved performance through health and nutrition. To control insulin, it is imperative that the intake of sugar is controlled and that refined carbohydrates are cut down to a minimum.

Avoiding refined carbohydrates results in lower average insulin levels in the blood throughout any given period. This has a markedly beneficial effect on reducing fat synthesis and storage, along with mitigating other adverse influences that insulin has on the cardiovascular system.

Again, it is emphasized that it is refined carbohydrates that do the damage; unrefined carbohydrates, however, require more digestive breakdown. And are, as a result, more slowly absorbed. The slower absorption modulates insulin secretion, reduces peaks in blood sugar concentration, and results in less fat synthesis and storage. So, consequently, there is less weight gain.

The Sugar Busters diet does not ban all carbohydrates! There is a particular emphasis on avoiding refined sugars. Many diets advocate eliminating almost all fat and meat, especially red meat. However, most people do not eat too much fat. All in all, some fat in the diet is necessary to synthesize steroids, lipoproteins, and other substances. These substances are essential for the proper metabolic operations of the body. Ingested fat plays a small role in excessive fat accumulation in the body.

Most of the excessive fat is due to the conversion of ingested carbohydrates to fat. Proponents of the Sugar Busters diet place great emphasis on the eating of meat. Ingested protein stimulates glucagon secretion, as well as providing the building blocks for the body. Glucagon promotes the breakdown of stored fat and helps counteract the effects of high insulin levels on the cardiovascular system.

With the Sugar Busters diet, alcohol, in reasonable amounts, is considered beneficial. Alcohol increases HDL cholesterol and decreases platelet stickiness and aggregation. This can lead to vascular thrombosis. These actions tend to reduce the development of arteriosclerosis and are likely to be achieved when red wine rather than other forms of alcohol is ingested.

Numerous studies illustrate that the number of deaths from cancer, heart disease, strokes, and accidents is cumulatively reduced in people who take one or two alcoholic beverages per day. However, not more than three: those who drink more than three run a higher risk of death from all causes and are particularly prone to liver disease. The consumption of alcohol remains somewhat controversial. And views are highly conflicting and range between complete extremes.

The proponents of the Sugar Busters diet place emphasis on eating patterns. Multiple meals stimulate less overall insulin secretion than one or two large feedings. Long periods of fasting alter the body's response to insulin by forcing it to enter conservation mode. This increases fat storage. It is therefore recommended that we strive to consume three balanced meals every day.

Sugar Busters expresses concern over eating too much fat, especially saturated fats. With multiple meals per day, portion size and control are very important. The portions of food selected for each meal should fit on the bottom of the plate and must not extend over the sides.

Second and third helpings are actively discouraged. It is beneficial to consume calories early in the day. Also, the consumption of large meals late at night is forbidden. Ingested cholesterol, it is thought, leads to elevations in serum cholesterol and the deposition of cholesterol into the arterial system.

Between meals, snacks should consist of fruits with the exception of watermelons, pineapples, raisins, and bananas. Why? Because all of them have a high glycemic index. This is a little surprising for watermelons, but it's a fact. Fruits contain the basic sugar fructose and stimulate approximately one-third of the insulin secretion that is secreted by glucose; consequently, fruit alone as a snack is beneficial.

Taken in combination with other carbohydrates, it loses the advantage of lowering insulin secretion that is achieved when eaten by itself. Fruits should be eaten whole. At the same time, fruit juices are discouraged because they inevitably contain a large amount of sugar.

Sugar Busters recommends consuming fluids between and particularly before meals as opposed to at the time of eating. They discourage the overconsumption of regular coffee and tea as a result of the caffeine stimulus. This can, in fact, interfere with sleep. Caffeine also makes the stomach secrete more acid, which stimulates appetite and might upset the stomach.

Drinking water throughout the day will discourage the desire to eat food, thereby helping weight control. Breakfast cereals are discouraged. Most breakfast cereals are laced with either white sugar, brown sugar, molasses, corn syrup, or honey. As a matter of fact, it is difficult to purchase pure natural grain cereal. Cereals based on oats are the healthiest. Furthermore, wheat bread is allowed in the form of whole grain rather than wholemeal.

SUGAR BUSTERS DIET

This is somewhat more liberal with carbohydrates than the Atkins diet. Banned carbohydrates are:

- Potatoes
- Corn
- White rice
- White bread
- Beets
- Carrots
- Granulated sugar
- Corn syrup
- Molasses
- Honey
- Sodas
- Beer

The Sugar Busters diet is thus aimed at reducing insulin secretion while enhancing the secretion of glucagon. The ultimate effect is a reduction of body fat and cholesterol, along with the many other health problems created by both.

Adequate sources of protein are a must! Forms of lean meat, such as beef, fish, and fowl, are recommended. These food items should have the fat removed and should be grilled, baked, or broiled, since frying involves the use of saturated fats.

Other excellent healthy protein sources are eggs and nuts, with possibly a little cheese. However, not too much of the latter as it is heavy in calories and fat. The proponents of this diet use the aphorism of “lighting the grill and throwing away the frying pan.”

Sugar Busters claimed to be creating a new nutritional lifestyle and a new form of healthy individual. It is logical, practical, and reasonable. It aims at removing unnecessary fat, especially saturated fat, from the diet. And thus, concentrating on the ingestion of lean and trimmed meats.

Refined carbohydrates are strictly forbidden, but starches may be taken in moderation. The Sugar Busters diet is a useful guide to a weight loss program. It is healthy and safe. Yet, it does not need to be pursued in the long term once the normal weight range has been achieved. And further advice on one's day-to-day diet will be discussed later.

It is clear from the above that the Sugar Busters and South Beach diets encompass almost exactly similar principles, strongly warning of the toxicity of eating excess sugar. Both of these diets are efficient in promoting weight loss. And in the end, it is down to individual preference as to which of these to adhere to. Or, in other words, form a combination of the two, employing the main underlying principles for each.

THE ATKINS DIET

The Atkins diet was claimed by the late author to be an easy-to-stay-with system that combines nutrition and vita nutrient supplements to a unique, weight-reducing, age-defying program. Atkins claimed that this diet added many years to life, boosted the immune defenses, and enhanced brain function and memory. It was also claimed that it reduces the risk of cardiovascular disease, permits weight loss without calorie restriction, and combats adult-onset diabetes.

The long-term assessment of the outcomes of this diet put into question some of Atkins' initial premises. These include a reduction of cardiovascular disease, which may, in fact, be increased by the diet. Atkins promulgated his diet against strong opposition from bodies such as the American Heart Association. The association has faced immense recent criticism regarding the strategy that they were promoting for the last half a century.

The Atkins diet involves a radical reduction of intake of carbohydrates. The only carbohydrates that are allowed are the complex and unrefined ones, basically starchy foods, including whole grains and lentils. Table sugar, sweets, cakes, cookies, and soft drinks are banned. These latter foods all have a high glycemic index that sends insulin levels and blood sugar concentrations soaring. Simple carbohydrates should be no more than 3% of the total diet. Pasta, bread, white rice, baked goods, candy, and soda are forbidden.

Atkins promotes little restriction on the ingestion of fats. He points out, however, that trans fats are the dietary link to elevated cholesterol and heart disease. Trans fats lower the good HDL cholesterol and raise the bad LDL cholesterol and the lipoproteins. Trans fats also reduce responsiveness to insulin and the uptake of essential fatty acids. He also emphasizes the use of safe food products with the avoidance of animal foods that contain antibiotics or hormones. He advocates the consumption of a wide spectrum of foods. These food items supply an array of vital nutrients and phytochemicals. They also avoid any chances for addiction to a specific foodstuff or produce, and vitamin and mineral deficiencies.

The first objective of the Atkins diet was to stabilize blood sugar concentrations, as is the case with the previous two diets discussed. This again is achieved by eliminating most simple carbohydrates and sugar-containing foods and replacing them with other complex carbohydrates or non-carbohydrate foods.

The Atkins diet allows complex carbohydrates, bans trans fats, recommends foods high in antioxidants, and allows fresh vegetables and some fruits.

Allows:

- All meats and fish
- Butter and some margarines
- Cheese and milk
- Oils and avocado
- Green vegetables
- Low-sugar fruits
- Atkins diet bans:
- All refined carbohydrates
- Sugar
- Sodas
- Cakes
- Cookies
- Canned fruits
- Drinks allowed in the Atkins diet:
- Eight 8-ounce glasses of water per day are encouraged
- Teas
- Coffee
- Diet sodas only
- Red wine

A convenience of the Atkins diet is that it is difficult to overeat if you adhere to the correct food items. Without refined carbohydrates, satiety is produced earlier. Unfortunately, ketones tend to be produced. And they can create headaches, fatigue, bad breath, and constipation. But they rarely build up to any significant degree.

The diet is based on a much higher-than-normal fat and protein content. And it is certainly much higher than that which is promoted with the South Beach or Sugar

Busters diet. A second objective of this diet is to create an intake of foods low in oxygen-free radicals and high in antioxidants that fight them. To increase antioxidant capacity, the diet is very high in fresh vegetables and low-sugar fruits such as berries.

An advantage of the diet is that, with those previously discussed, the patient does not have to count calories or even excessively restrict portion size. Atkins stated that steak and fish may be eaten with free access to fresh vegetables. Brown rice and whole grain bread are allowed.

Some cheeses are permitted. Yet, yogurts, which are high in lactose, a simple sugar, should be kept to a minimum. Bran is allowed, and nuts and seeds are encouraged. Atkins recommended taking butter rather than margarine, stating that margarines contain large amounts of trans fats that release cascades of artery-damaging free radicals. This is somewhat controversial! Remember that butter and margarine are very high in calories. However, fat intake helps to stabilize blood sugar concentrations.

Recommended are the monounsaturated vegetable oils such as olive, almond, avocado, and macadamia. These oils are excellent sources of omega-3 and omega-6 fatty acids. The consumption of complex carbohydrates is allowed as these are more likely to maintain the blood sugar at a steady level. This is especially the case when combined with protein and fat.

Generous and varied portions of salad greens, broccoli, kale, Brussels sprouts, and green vegetables are encouraged. Potatoes are again frowned upon. Vegetables are better than fruits; the latter should only be taken in moderation. Fruits are a good source of fiber, vitamins, minerals, and other essential nutrients. However, fruits contain ample amounts of simple carbohydrates and fruit juices, which have added sugars and are to be avoided at all costs.

Canned fruits have virtually no nutritional value and are loaded with added sugar. And thus, they should be avoided. The drinking of tea is allowed with no restrictions. However, Atkins discourages coffee consumption in contrast to the previous two diets discussed. Other nutritionists have in recent years become stronger advocates of coffee. Alcoholic beverages may again be taken in moderation. Beer and dessert wines, however, should be avoided.

Choices among fruits or berries are of any kind, but frozen berries frequently have added sugar. A cup of blueberries, which are the best of all the berries, contains about 10g of carbohydrates. This amounts to only 40 calories.

Avocados are an excellent source of monounsaturated fat and are, therefore, a healthy fat. It has been stated recently that carotenoids such as lycopene may help to prevent cancer, particularly cancer of the prostate. This remains somewhat questionable. And lycopene has been added to many of the over-the-counter vitamin preparation products. Sources of these are dark green leafy vegetables and carrots, with high concentrations being present in tomatoes.

A disadvantage of the Atkins diet is that with such a somewhat extreme reduction in carbohydrates, the body does not burn fat efficiently and produces compounds called ketones. Ketones accumulate in the blood. These sometimes cause nausea, headache, fatigue, bad breath, and constipation. They can put a strain on the kidneys. There is some debate now as to whether this diet increases the risk of heart disease, vascular disease, and even cancer due to its relatively high concentration of fats.

Ironically, perhaps, the diet has been shown to be associated with lower levels of serum cholesterol, which is a surprise. Overall, the Atkins diet is now dated; it was the forerunner of the sugar-free diets. However, it has been superseded by the two previously discussed low-carbohydrate diets. These are to be preferred over the more extreme Atkins diet. The question of an increased risk of heart disease remains, which is what Atkins himself died from; it is therefore advised not to adhere strictly to the Atkins diet.

HIGH PROTEIN DIETS

The Eades diet is essentially a low-carbohydrate diet that depends upon the rationale of eating large amounts of protein to improve lean body mass but not to stimulate insulin, and therefore, the overall effect is a slimmer, healthier body. It is also encouraged for people to eat only a small amount of fat. This is quite probably a good diet for athletes and weightlifters, but it is expensive. High protein drinks such as "Lean Body" contain a large amount of protein, up to 40g in a single 300mL drink, and relatively small amounts of carbohydrate. These drinks are good and are recommended.

It has recently been claimed by two Australian academics at the University of Sydney that if you eat too little protein, you will be tormented by cravings. And as a result, likely to overindulge in all the wrong foods. All the while, on a high-protein diet, your appetite can be satisfied with fewer calories. It is claimed that if you eat a plate of fish or chicken, you won't be tempted to go on to eating foods that are predominantly fat and carbohydrates. The higher protein intake will help us to build muscle and produce enzymes for growth, cell replacement, and repair.

We eat too much ultra-processed food, lacking in protein. And this results in obesity, which must be avoided at all costs. Eating eggs or fish for breakfast rather than carbohydrate-laden cereals and bread ensures that hunger and calorie consumption will be reduced later in the day.

It was discovered by the late Dr. Michael Mosley that when hunger strikes, you should drink a cup of plain tea or coffee, up to four cups per day. He recommended planning activities or exercise programs to avoid key craving trigger points in the day. We should aim to get 15 to 20% of our calories from protein to avoid pangs of hunger. This means eating a minimum of 45g for women and 55g for men. As you get older, you need more protein. A medium-sized egg contains 8g of protein and provides about 80 calories.

WEIGHT WATCHERS (WW)

A popular diet that has a huge following is the Weight Watchers diet. This, in some ways, might seem to fly in the face of the principles outlined above that underlie the strategy for the other more popular weight-reducing diets. Whatever the confab, the Weight Watchers diet is successful for many people.

Moreover, a large amount of weight can be lost by following their principles. This diet has been around for many years, and the company has gone through multiple ownerships with many radical changes. It employs a totally different philosophy, strategically based on a points system. The subject is restricted to staying within a fixed number of points daily. It does not conduct a calorie count, as such. And most points allocated are perhaps surprising. But, again, the system does work!

There are no restrictions on the foods that you can eat, provided that you do not exceed the daily points limit, which has both a maximum and a minimum. Weight Watchers offers as many as 8,000 recipes for program participants to choose from.

Some food items are surprisingly classed as scoring no points. Though obviously, they contain calories. Examples are skinless chicken, turkey breast, fish, shellfish, and even eggs. Two slices of bread are, however, three points, a Big Mac counts 18 points, one cup of whole milk is seven points, and a foot-long Subway American Club contains 32 points.

Some of the foods listed as freestyle—no points—are the following: apples, beans, broccoli, coleslaw, eggs, mushrooms, onions, salads, and mixed vegetables. You can eat as much of these as you like. Although many aspects of the Weight Watchers diet seem to contradict the principles used in strict calorie-restricted enforcement, the system does work and has been beneficial to many thousands, at least in the short term. Part of the strategy is to encourage participants to regularly attend meetings, almost like the 12 steps.

It must be said that most diets in the long term ultimately fail; this is largely because people tend to stray away from the restrictions of their diets. And, ultimately, while becoming disillusioned, they return to their old bad habits.

It has recently been reported that more than 2,000 diabetics, with Type 2 diabetes, put on a regimen of soup and shakes to reverse diabetes, lost an average of 30 pounds in just three months. Previous studies have found that half of the people with Type 2 diabetes can reverse the condition if they adhere to strict diets for several months. A diet that reduces calories to about 800 a day, provided that they maintain their weight loss in the long term.

Further studies are being carried out on over 10,000 people. This study was targeted at those aged between 18 and 65, with a body mass index of over 27. And also those who had a Type 2 diabetes diagnosis for at least six years and were of Black, Asian, or minority ethnic origin. These people are those at the highest risk for diabetes and its complications.

All of the above diets I have described place emphasis on drinking large amounts of water: many at least eight glasses per day, or calorie-free drinks, which in itself is not easy to achieve. Fruits and vegetables contain a large amount of water. But basically, all of the essential vitamins and minerals are required for good health.

LONGEVITY

It has long been known that there are groups of people in the world who live extraordinarily long lives while maintaining good health throughout. These long-living people are the Abkhazians of Russia, the Vicabans of Ecuador, and the Hunzakuts of Pakistan. There is no obesity in these societies. And they all live amazingly disease-free lives without apparent heart or vascular disease. It is claimed that there is neither cancer nor any heart disease prevalent in their society. Their diet is essentially comprised of fruits and vegetables.

I am not trying to advocate that you live your lives firmly attached to any of these diets, which are principally designed to achieve weight loss. But they all, in their various ways, illustrate what is involved in healthy eating and what foods should be avoided. They are all based on the underlying principle that refined carbohydrates are bad for you. And also the fact that these are the major causes of all the diseases killing us in present-day society.

CHAPTER 14: EARLY APPETITE SUPPRESSANT DRUGS IN THE MANAGEMENT OF THE OBESE PATIENT

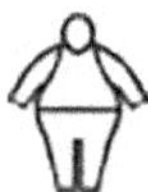

Over the years, many appetite suppressants have been used, especially fenfluramine, phentermine, and mazindol. All of these appetite suppressants, in the short term, lessen hunger and possibly decrease food intake in normal-weight subjects.

Fenfluramine was withdrawn by the FDA about a decade ago as a result of its tendency to cause pulmonary hypertension, or lung damage. These symptoms occurred in a small number of individuals treated with this drug. These drugs are also stimulants that tend to increase metabolic rate. However, they have largely been used in appetite suppression. Yet, their efficacy has always been open to question, and they are now less commonly used.

EARLY APPETITE SUPPRESSANT DRUGS

The majority of placebo-controlled double-blind clinical trials of appetite suppressant drugs used in the management of obesity have shown a significantly greater loss of weight. Even though not impressively so, in those patients receiving the active drug rather than the placebo. The effect on the whole has most noticeably been seen in the first four weeks of treatment, and thereafter, weight loss has decreased.

Few trials of these early drugs have demonstrated continuing weight loss after periods of three to six months. Moreover, after stopping drug therapy, a large proportion of the weight lost has been regained. Sometimes, more is gained than lost. There is also a risk of drug dependency and drug abuse with these agents. And unfortunately, they are frequently related to amphetamines. However, total dependence is unusual. And the majority of obese patients find little difficulty in stopping these drugs.

Use of these early appetite suppressant drugs has, on the whole, been limited to those who have a substantial risk to physical or mental health as a result of the obese state. Even so, in the morbidly obese, the maximal weight loss has not been impressive. Drugs may act in part as an adjunct to dieting or behavioral therapy. A combination of these modalities is immensely beneficial in the short term. The sudden withdrawal of the drugs can sometimes lead to overt depressive symptoms.

Most of these weight-reducing drugs stimulate the sympathetic nervous system. And therefore, side effects erupt like insomnia, restlessness, irritability, dry mouth, and tachycardia, or rapid heartbeat. They should not be used in patients with angina. Commonly reported adverse effects also include nausea and diarrhea.

The first drug that was widely used in the treatment of obesity was phentermine, which was introduced in the late 1950s. Phentermine was combined with a drug called "topiramate," and the combination of these drugs suppressed appetite. The topiramate component was originally mainly used singly to treat seizures, migraine, and headaches. The combination of these drugs was contraindicated in patients with glaucoma, hyperthyroidism, and pregnancy.

In the 1970s, fenfluramine also became available, and these drugs were widely used in combination under the name "Fen/Phen." In the late 1990s, it became apparent that they could be associated with cardiorespiratory problems. And in consequence, they were withdrawn from the market. Prior to their withdrawal, some 14 million prescriptions were written for these drugs each year.

Sibutramine (Meridia) is an appetite suppressant reported to give a sensation of early satiety. Studies have shown a weight loss of about 10% of the starting weight at the end of one year. The drug is a stimulant and can increase blood pressure and cardiac rate; thus, significant concerns have existed tied to its use, particularly in the elderly.

Other drugs that have been used as appetite suppressants are Tenuate Dospan, Didrax, Bontirl, and Adipex. None of these agents has been FDA-approved for the treatment of obesity, and the results of their use have been unimpressive. The antidepressants Prozac, Zoloft, and Wellbutrin have been widely used in weight loss programs, though their established role is in the treatment of depressive illnesses.

Topamax is a drug that has found some success. It is fundamentally an anticonvulsant but also works to some extent as an appetite suppressant, sometimes causing impressive weight loss. Metformin, a drug used in the treatment of Type 2 diabetes, is thought to promote a more efficient use of glucose. It may also be effective in producing a small amount of weight loss, particularly in Type 2 diabetics. An antidepressant, which is available over the counter as a nutraceutical, is St. John's wort. This drug seems to work like a mild SSRI-type antidepressant.

A drug that has a totally different mode of action is Orlistat. This drug blocks the absorption of fat from the intestinal tract. Side effects of diarrhea, abdominal pain, and liver damage have been reported. Patients should take a multivitamin preparation, particularly a fat-absorption vitamin, to correct impaired fat absorption produced by the drug. In a large study carried out by the European Obesity Study Group, this drug, which had been administered for two years, was shown to promote weight loss, minimize weight regain, and improve lipid profile, blood pressure, and quality of life.

Diarrhea from the malabsorption of fat is a side effect of the use of this drug. The pharmaceutical companies—being well aware of the great potential that exists for an efficacious form of drug therapy—are currently carrying out a large number of clinical trials on new agents.

Many clinical trials for prescription medications have been carried out and are being increasingly investigated. The overriding questions relating to these preliminary drugs are how much weight can be lost, what the side effects are, how long the patients have to stay on the drug, and whether the drug interacts with existing medications. And, more importantly, what is the relapse rate because the latter tends to be very high? Finally, these drugs must be combined with an effective, healthy, long-term, tolerable diet.

Other drugs referred to as "fat burners" are also claimed to boost energy and mental focus. L-tyrosine and caffeine have been advocated. Juniper berry extract and white willow bark are said to be effective. The combination of these drugs, called DMHA drugs, has been available for decades and contains natural ingredients. It has been claimed that they suppress appetite and increase metabolism.

High doses of caffeine can cause anxiety and nervousness. Contrave is a substance that, it is claimed, targets two areas of the brain that are responsible for feelings of hunger and cravings. The FDA approved them, and moderate weight loss has been achieved in several studies, including 2,322 patients.

Contrave can cause serious side effects, including suicidal thoughts or actions. One of the ingredients is the antidepressant bupropion, which may be most dangerous in vulnerable teenagers. Irritability, aggression, and anger may occur. It should not be taken by patients who are hypotensive. Seizures have also been reported with bupropion.

Few patients treated with these older drugs reach their goal weight, and almost none reach their ideal weight. Previously available drugs helped to produce a mean weight loss of about 10% of body weight at the start of treatment, but there is a high relapse rate. As obesity is a chronic, usually lifelong condition, the value of the established drugs has been very limited. And till now, no "best drug" has emerged from these early medications.

CHAPTER 15: AN EXCITING NEW THERAPEUTIC DEVELOPMENT THAT COULD POTENTIALLY CHANGE THE PLAYING FIELD

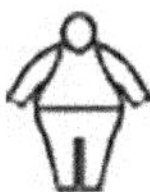

NEW AND EFFECTIVE DRUGS WEGOVY

Very recently, a number of new drugs which belong to the category of semaglutides—produced by Novo Nordisk—of which the major ones are Wegovy and Ozempic, the latter has been developed largely for the management of Type 2 diabetes. Wegovy has recently been developed for adults with morbid obesity and weight-related medical problems, used with reduced-calorie meal plans and increased physical activity.

In a 60-week duration medical study of 1,961 adults living with obesity or excess weight who had a related medical problem, the drug was used with reduced calorie intake and increased physical activity. Spectacular results were achieved: adults with an average starting weight of 232 pounds achieved a 35-pound weight loss, 15% of their initial weight. This was compared to a placebo drug, where people lost an average of six pounds, 2.5% of their initial body weight.

The people in this study treated with Wegovy kept their weight off while they continued to take the drug. Eighty-two percent of adults taking Wegovy lost weight compared to 31% taking a placebo. More than 10% of the initial weight was lost by 66% of those taking Wegovy, compared to 12% taking a placebo. And more than 15% of initial body weight was lost by those taking Wegovy compared with 5% taking a placebo. One in three adults lost more than 46 pounds, 20% of the initial weight, while taking the drug. In a supportive measure to this study, 30% taking Wegovy lost 20% or more of their body weight compared to only 2% of the placebo-treated group.

The BMI of patients in this study was over 30. And of those with weight-related problems, including hypertension and elevated cholesterol, all had a BMI of over 27. Patients with Type 2 diabetes were excluded from this study. Instructions were given to all participants to adhere to a reduced-calorie meal plan and increased physical activity. This was the same for both the active and placebo-treated groups. Seven percent of people taking Wegovy (92 people) left the study due to side effects of the drug compared with 3.1% of people taking the placebo (20 people). Wegovy is an injectable semaglutide given in a recommended dosage of 2.4mg.

There are a number of other semaglutide drugs. Mounjaro (tirzepatide) is said to produce similar results and is manufactured in Mexico. Trulicity (dulaglutide), Rabelis, and Saxenda (liraglutide) have also been developed. There has been a massive demand for these drugs. And the Scandinavian manufacturers are unable to provide them to all potential purchasers.

These drugs have been shown, in a small minority, to cause serious side effects, including thyroid tumors, and rarely thyroid cancer. The patients can be alerted to this by identifying a lump or swelling in the neck, hoarseness, trouble swallowing, or shortness of breath. There may be symptoms of thyroid cancer in addition.

Studies in rodents have shown the development of thyroid tumors, including cancers. There is as yet no evidence that Wegovy can cause a type of thyroid cancer called medullary thyroid cancer (MTC), nor has Multiple Endocrine Neoplasia, Type 2 (MEN 2) been reported.

Anyone with a history of thyroid cancer or MEN 2 should not take these drugs. Also, rare cases of serious allergic reactions have occurred. Other contraindications are pancreatic or kidney disease, diabetic retinopathy, depression or suicidal thoughts, pregnancy, or breastfeeding. It is important for patients to report to their physician all other medicines They are taking vitamins, herbal supplements, diabetic medications, including sulfonylureas or insulin.

Part of the reasoning why Wegovy reduces weight is that it slows gastric emptying, which might affect the absorption of foodstuffs. Pancreatitis—manifested by upper abdominal pain radiating through to the back—can occur and is an indication for the abrupt cessation of the drug. The development of gallstones has also been reported. This may necessitate surgical treatment.

In diabetics, hypoglycemia may occur, particularly in patients on sulfonylureas or insulin. Symptoms of low blood sugar may occur and are manifested by dizziness, blurred vision, lightheadedness, anxiety, irritability, shakiness, weakness, headache, and confusion.

Kidney problems may result from dehydration, nausea, and vomiting. It is important to drink water with the treatment. Rash, itching, facial pain, or throat swelling indicates an allergic reaction, which can be severe. Seizures have also been reported.

The current situation, rest between a long-term assessment of the efficacy of the new semaglutide drugs, and the outcomes of surgery. This includes side effects and the safety of the optimal surgical procedures, gastric bypass and gastric sleeve resection, along with their potential complications.

Pfizer has a new oral semaglutide (danuglipron). This has been claimed to produce the same amount of weight loss as Wegovy and Ozempic. In fact, a study was recently published in JAMA in May 2023.

The appetite suppressive effects of all of the injected semaglutides kick in after a few days and persist throughout the course of the treatment. There is a loss of appetite and sometimes a bloated sensation, with occasionally a feeling of chills. Food cravings disappear, and the desire for fat, sugar, and salt goes.

Emphasis is placed on firm adherence to a dietary intake of simple foods with increased vegetables, white meat, and avoidance of refined carbohydrates. Dietary advice is strongly recommended and should be insisted upon. There is a definite need to eat healthy foods, not just to reduce overall calorie intake. The need for essential proteins, fatty acids, vitamins, and minerals, as reiterated consistently, is mandatory. The dietary recommendations outlined earlier in this book underlie diet usage with the semaglutides. There are no known dietary idiosyncrasies related to these drugs.

As outlined above, not only are weight losses of 60 to 70 pounds with a harvesting of excess body fat achievable in the first six months. However, diabetes is completely controlled, and high blood pressure is reduced. Claims of a reduced occurrence of cancer and dementia have been made. But only with increased time and observation can these be accurately determined. A reduction of stress has also been trained with a possible positive personality change.

Somewhat improved results have been achieved with Mounjaro over Wegovy, but these can be dose-dependent. Ozempic is an excellent drug for the control of diabetes. But it is less effective than Wegovy in producing weight loss. In a short-term comparative study, Mounjaro produced a mean 22% weight loss and regularly at the same time achieved 15%.

These powerful drugs are expensive. But the cost of treating heart disease, diabetes, stroke, dementia, and osteoarthritis of the hips and knees is hundreds of billions of dollars each year. In the UK, Wegovy and Mounjaro are available on the NHS. It is estimated that in the UK alone, 4 million people could be eligible for treatment with these drugs.

These people would need to have a BMI of over 40, together with several comorbidities. It has been stated, however, that anyone with a BMI of 27 or more would benefit from semaglutide. It is rumored that some may purposely increase their weight in order to qualify for treatment. A significant requirement is that patients on these drugs are regularly followed up by a medical practitioner. Despite the vast cost of the drugs, it has been estimated that their use could potentially save millions in the healthcare budget.

The use of these drugs could overcome the need for bariatric surgery, the risks and side effects of which are greater than those of the medication. Given the choice, it is likely that the vast majority of patients would prefer to receive semaglutide rather than undergo the major types of surgery described herein.

In addition, most patients following surgery in the long term regain a considerable amount of weight that they had lost. However, the cessation of the semaglutide will almost inevitably result in further weight gain. The duration of treatment with the summer glue tied could even need to be lifelong.

The demand for these drugs is huge. And the major problem has arisen with their illicit production and marketing from China to scam sales sources in the US and the UK. The *Daily Mail* in June 2025 published that *Cheap Do it Yourself Ozempic* is being sold in a blooming black market that puts life at risk.

Dealers are using social media to openly advertise their cut-price illegal fat jabs to vulnerable people without legally required medical supervision. The genuine drugs are made by Novo Nordisk, who own the patents for Wegovy and Ozempic, and Eli Lilly owns the patent for Mounjaro. A flourishing trade of centers producing counterfeit versions of these drugs has sprung up in China, from where they are distributed widely. Many of these drugs are dispatched to patients using Facebook.

Warnings have been widely distributed that these drugs—as sold on social media—pose a very serious risk to health, and deaths have occurred. When legitimately purchased, the drugs cost about $300 per month. It is imperative that these drugs are prescribed only by legitimate physicians, and careful follow-up, sometimes with dose adjustments, is crucial. There remain important issues to be addressed: the cost of the drugs, the dose regulation, and the duration of treatment.

CHAPTER 16: BEHAVIORAL THERAPY

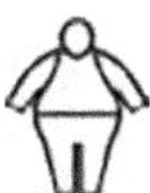

Behavioral techniques are often based on close monitoring and peer pressure. They frequently involve keeping a record of every food and drink item consumed and all physical activities. Programs are often individually tailored to suit personality and lifestyle. Self-help groups frequently play a vital role in this kind of therapy. And often, mentors are available at any time to assist when the patient is experiencing difficulty.

The detailed documentation of the patient's eating habits and exercise forms an important base of self-education. This can then be manipulated appropriately. Once the principal elements underlying the subject's behavior have been established, certain disciplines are involved. The patient is advised to sit down for all meals, adhere to a fixed time-controlled eating regimen, eat slowly, avoid snacks, and drink plenty of water. They are advised to resist the temptation to purchase inappropriate food items for the home.

Weighing of the subjects takes place about once every two weeks. Peer group meetings are frequently held. Peer pressure is an important stimulus for the patient to adhere to the program. The most widely known system that adheres to this sort of philosophy is "Weight Watchers."

Boredom and inactivity are common reasons for eating. Those who are engaged in stimulating and creative mental activity are much less likely to snack while working. If, however, calories are restricted to too great an extent, then the subject becomes increasingly focused on eating. The way around this is to eat celery, drink water, or stop working and take frequent walks.

Some individuals eat excessively when under stress. It has been shown that obese women are more emotionally reactive. And hence, more likely to engage in emotional eating than women of normal weight. The more emotional the women feel, the more likely they are to eat to achieve solace.

A common feature noticed among obese people is that, when in company, they eat either the same amount as others or even sometimes markedly less. In contrast, when alone, they tend to binge eat. Behavioral therapy focuses on dealing with the emotional factors that affect eating.

Other ways of overcoming an intense desire to eat are by making a phone call to friends to relieve loneliness and anxiety or by sending an email to someone who has a similar problem. Obesity leads to social isolation. And that, in itself, is a motivator for eating for several people. Being dissatisfied with one's own weight is a factor that predisposes to the above conditions and can be a stimulus to eating.

Surveys of women have shown that while most women are self-conscious about some aspect of their appearance, most focus their attention on their weight. And more than 80% of women claim that they would like to be slimmer. This situation has been accentuated by the modern tendency to choose extremely thin women as fashion models.

These thin women are often bordering on anorexia. The ideal shape of a woman as manifested by art and advertising can be illustrated by the change. This has occurred from the time of Rubens and Rembrandt, where women were voluptuous. In the 1950s, the ideal was portrayed by Marilyn Monroe. In contrast, in the present day, Calvin Klein underwear advertisements reveal only skin and bone! The same, to some extent, is true for men. This is where models are usually tall and thin but muscular.

Society dictates how people should look. And, in reality, achieving these ideals is difficult or impossible, at least for most. The inability to achieve them might be associated with failure, giving rise to people either opting out of the race. Or, as a result of the anxiety it produces, overeating is considered a rebound phenomenon.

Controlled clinical trials of behavioral therapy have shown that patients lose about 10 pounds in the first eight to 10 weeks. During that time, compliance tends to be good, and dropout rates are low. With increasing periods of time, however, many members abandon the program. And the overall maintenance of weight loss beyond one year is extremely rare. A large study of behavioral therapy programs showed that 16% maintained their weight loss of over 40 pounds, and 17% were heavier than at the start of the program.

People investing in behavioral treatments, therefore, can expect to achieve results perhaps as good as, if not better than, those which are achieved by the older forms of drug therapy. The results of both of these treatment modalities, in the long term, however, are very disappointing. No one has adequately addressed the problem of long-term maintenance!

Systems of rewards have been used, and these appear only to be valuable in the short term. Similarly, the use of penalties appears to be inefficient over time. Perhaps the most important adjunct to this form of therapy is social support. And with close interdependence, results tend to be better.

Some people in these behavioral programs are able to communicate instantly by email in the hope of gaining help and overcoming the tendency to depart from the strict constraints of the program. Studies have shown that individual treatment by a therapist produces better results than group therapy alone. Although behavioral therapy is designed to provide a set of skills to identify and modify inappropriate eating, stimulate exercise, and good thinking habits, these programs most frequently end in failure, and the lost weight is completely regained.

Another form of therapy that could broadly be included under the heading of behavioral is psychiatric management. Society is geared to the ingestion of calorie-dense food. There has been a portion size inflation. And foods of high fat and carbohydrate content are the most heavily advertised products on television.

Moreover, obesity leads to depression. And as we know, depression is commonly associated with binge eating or snacking to achieve solace. Psychiatric management combines with cognitive therapy. An overall eating plan may be used to instruct the patients in the basics of nutrition. Drugs are frequently used as an adjunct to this form of therapy. Psychotherapy plays a role, and support contact through email is also advocated.

Individuals are motivated by different factors. One patient who lost 130 pounds did so because she became frustrated on a hike with her teenage daughter. The woman was so breathless after walking a short distance that she had to sit down on a bench. An elderly man with a cane passed her by, as did a person in a wheelchair. This was the straw that broke the camel's back.

It was that image that she kept in her mind every time she was tempted by things like a plate of cookies or some high-calorie food. She would repeat to herself, "If this is going to stop my chances of hiking with my daughter, it's not worth it."

Other patients are similarly motivated by discovering that they are unable to get into the clothes they wish to buy. Similarly, they see that the clothes that do fit them are either hard to obtain or singularly unattractive. Conversely, some are loath to go on diets because they feel they will never be able to eat their favorite foods again. This is far from the truth! Specially designed diets exist that can incorporate favorite foods without resulting in excess calorie intake, provided the overall balance is good.

A good rule of thumb is the 80-20 rule. About 80% of foods eaten should be lean protein. These include food items, poultry, fish, and beans, fruits and vegetables, low-fat dairy such as skim milk, high-fiber grain products, and healthier fats such as olive oil. The other 20% of the time, they can eat foods that are not so helpful.

No one is saying weight loss is easy; it takes a lot of work, a long time, and may even be expensive. It is hard to change lifelong habits. And even harder to purchase different foods that have to be prepared in various ways. Habits that are sometimes more expensive than those previously bought. It is financially viable in the long term by reducing the obesity-associated morbidity that will inevitably accrue.

CHAPTER 17: BEHAVIORAL THERAPY: SHOULD YOU JOIN A GROUP?

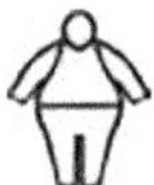

Behavioral therapy programs depend, sometimes greatly, upon the effects of peer pressure. They offer differing disciplines underlying the strategy for weight loss. However, all involve group meetings, where participants compare results and share problems. The atmosphere is one that creates commitments and applies pressure in order for the patient to achieve the desired results. Patients can often choose the approach that suits them best. Approaches often depend upon calorie counting, but "no counting plans."

Programs vary in terms of group size and number of visits required. Some of these programs not only spell out exact data requirements but also require the purchase of special meals. A number of these plans exist online, while others involve internet weight loss companionship for Weight Watchers meetings. These provide access to recipes and tools to people who are already attending meetings, allegedly making it easier to stay on the plan and appreciate progress.

Weight Watchers is among the largest plans and provides individualized diets, as mentioned above, which are based on a point system. There is flexibility in the choice of foods. And it is possible to earn extra points by exercising. However, it is imperative that the allocated number of points is not exceeded.

The Weight Watchers Flex Plan allows subjects to enjoy the full range of food options while making better choices within the confines of the point system. Any food can be chosen. The essential factor is being in control of how much is eaten. An alternative to the Flex Plan is the Core Plan. This plan focuses on wholesome foods without calorie counting. Patients are allowed to eat from a list of wholesome foods from all food groups. It is stated that they can enjoy satisfying eating without "empty calories." And at the same time, they are allowed an occasional treat in controlled amounts.

Weight Watchers' meetings provide coaching and insights in order to help subjects reach their goals. They are taught to make wise choices, eat healthily, and enjoy a combination of food and exercise. The support and guidance are major factors in enabling them to reach their goal and stay there.

Participants in the plan benefit from the practical experiences, tips, and peer pressure of others losing weight with the system. Along with the meeting, Weight Watchers online provides interactive resources encouraging following of the plan in a step-by-step way. Access to tips and strategies is provided to encourage following the plan. It is stated that this makes it easier to manage food choices and activities and discover many delicious recipes. Plus, the internet weight loss comparison gives email addresses for subjects to contact peers in times of need.

Weight Watchers' staff includes registered dietitians, exercise physiologists, and clinical psychologists. Lifetime members may become leaders who deliver the program to familiarize participants. The average cost of the Weight Watchers plan is a one-time registration fee of $20 with a weekly fee of $10–$15. If the subject is qualified for lifetime membership, then it becomes free. Some 20,000 meetings are held weekly within North America.

Patients are encouraged to attend meetings once per week for about one hour. There is no formal contact. As a result, fees are only paid for meetings attended. Each week, there is a confidential weigh-in to measure progress. Advice is given on making wise choices, eating healthily, and enjoying food and exercise. Every week, tips and new program materials are given.

The Weight Watchers program leader explains the strategy and identifies goals. Meeting leaders are usually people who have had successful outcomes from the program. They undergo formal training in these plans and are committed to the success and to their own maintenance of weight loss. Subjects also benefit from advice, recipes, and other experiences.

Members can sign up for Weight Watchers E-tools and online weight loss advice. Getting started is easy once the patient provides their personal address, and local meetings are identified online. And the atmosphere is altogether friendly and positive.

With the Flex Plan, subjects are given a points calculator and points tracker containing a list of over a thousand recipes and points value for each. A Flex Plan restaurant guide is given to provide advice when eating out. Access is available around the clock.

For the Core Plan, the patient is given a comprehensive core food list with all of the essential foods they can enjoy without tracking or counting. They can browse hundreds of core recipes, comprehensive items, and ideas. Success is charted on a weight tracker and progress chart, and a Core Plan restaurant guide exists.

The Jenny Craig program employs a philosophy-based, unexercised lifestyle modification and the taking of a low-calorie diet. Subjects are encouraged to eat three meals a day and three snacks. Much emphasis is placed on increased physical activity. Packaged foods are available and recommended, particularly during the early phases.

A weight loss of about one to two pounds per week is usually achieved, which is similar to the rate on Weight Watchers. However, the long-term results are not as good. The staff involved in the Jenny Craig program are registered dietitians who work with trained non-medical personnel. The latter have completed a training session and participate in regular updating educational sessions. The Jenny Craig program is more expensive than Weight Watchers.

Optifast is a medically supervised rapid weight loss program that is administered in hospitals and clinics. The plan requires liquid meal replacements and food bars. Dietary requirements are stringent, and participants are assigned to an 800, 950, or 1200-calorie package. This program is intended for those who are at least 50 pounds overweight. All the while, the program runs for approximately three months, followed by a six-month transitional period.

Emphasis is placed on increased physical activity, and individual counseling is available. It has already been pointed out that although physical activity is an extremely important adjunct to most weight loss programs, it does not in itself produce a large amount of weight loss. Individual counseling is available.

These programs are more expensive, often costing about $5000 for the whole program. Health management resources provide medically supervised rapid weight loss programs for patients who are 50 pounds or more overweight. Diets as low as 500 calories per day are provided, and these are monitored by medical personnel.

Meal replacements and special foods need to be purchased in order to adhere accurately to the requirements of the more radical programs. Weekly meetings are held. A weight loss of between 15 pounds a week is expected in the early days. It is frequently achieved with some tailing off thereafter. The programs are run by physicians, registered dietitians, nurses, and psychologists.

Some programs exist that place emphasis upon peer support but do not require a planned battery structure. The structure of the staff supervising these programs is based on the provision of psychologists and registered dietitians. Psychologists place emphasis on developing internal skills of self-nurturing and adhering to limits to achieve a diet that is free from excess. Tele-coaching is available through videoconference centers.

All of these programs work to some extent, particularly in the early stages, but program abandonment is common. And rebound weight gain is the norm. Most of these programs include physical activity recommendations, and emphasis is placed on the importance of adhering to these. Once again, there tends to be a considerable falloff in adherence to exercise programs.

Radical programs such as those which employ a diet of less than 1000 calories may be associated with certain health risks: an increased incidence of gallstones and their complications, or even coronary artery disease. Vitamin deficiencies may also develop. Cost is often an important factor in determining whether or not subjects participate in the more expensive range of available programs. The least expensive of these programs is Weight Watchers.

CHAPTER 18: TECHNIQUES USED IN SURGICALLY TREATING OBESITY

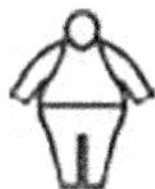

Surgical approaches to the problem of morbid obesity have existed for approximately 70 years. And the number of procedures has increased at a very rapid rate over recent years. The field was slow to gain acceptance in the early years. Why? Because obesity was considered by the vast majority not so much a disease but more of a consequence of a lack of self-control.

In recent years, it has become apparent that morbid obesity can rarely be reversed by diet alone or a simple change in lifestyle. It is now equally apparent that modern methods of surgical treatment can not only result in massive weight reduction but also in an amelioration of the life-threatening problems typically associated with the morbidly obese state.

TECHNIQUES USED IN THE SURGICAL TREATMENT OF OBESITY

- Resection of large lengths of the small intestine
- Jejunoileal bypass
- Jaw wiring
- Intragastric balloon
- Gastroplasty
- Vertical banded (ring) gastroplasty
- GASTRIC SLEEVE RESECTION

- ROUX–EN–Y GASTRIC BYPASS

The first operation for obesity was carried out in 1954. A long length of small intestine was taken out of the circuit and bypassed. This resulted in the patient's weight falling from 385 pounds at the time of surgery to stabilize at 140 pounds. This patient ultimately went on to undergo another batch of bypass surgery in 1971 and lost a further 50 pounds. The patient died in 1981 of a heart attack.

One patient had been reported in 1952, in whom a large amount of the small intestine was removed and not bypassed. And this resulted in considerable weight loss.

In the early 1960s, several different procedures were tried: the difference being the length of intestine which was left in the circuit. It became apparent that large amounts of weight could be lost by bypassing a major part of the small intestine. Between 1962 and 1975, there were trials of several different types of intestinal bypass.

JEJUNOILEAL BYPASS

These operations had various lengths of small intestine excluded, which left intact only 42 to 100 cm in the main intestinal tract. The bypassed small intestine was initially left in place and usually drained into the colon. The ultimate results, in terms of weight loss achieved with these procedures, were good. However, side effects were common, unpredictable, and often life-threatening. As a result, these procedures were later abandoned.

The various types of jejunoileal or small intestinal bypass produced differing amounts of weight loss. This was roughly related to the amount of intestine remaining in the circuit. With retained lengths longer than 100 cm, weight loss normally proved to be unsatisfactory.

With lengths shorter than 45 cm, the occurrence of protein malnutrition rose sharply. Some remarkable results were obtained from this operation, and long-term weight loss was sustained. However, the late complication of liver failure was especially alarming and led to some deaths. In addition, some patients developed electrolyte abnormalities in the blood. This can lead to cardiac arrhythmias and potential fatalities.

Kidney stones, arthritis, gallbladder disease, hernia, persistent diarrhea, and malnutrition with dehydration all occurred after these operations. Unfortunately, there was no way of predicting before surgery which patient was going to develop a malnourished state or any of the above complications.

Jejunoileal bypass was abandoned, partly because of the high rate of complications. There was also a significant number of patients who did not maintain their initial weight loss. And late weight gain after five to 10 years was common. The operation possibly gained a false adverse reaction to its outcome. Several people had a good long-term result; some forms of intestinal bypass remain in use today when combined with other procedures such as gastric reduction.

JAW WIRING

Another early procedure was dental occlusion or jaw wiring. In this procedure, the teeth are capped, and the jaws are wired in a fixed, slightly open position. It is impossible for the patient to take solid food, and a milk-based liquid diet is prescribed. In some patients, approximately 60% of the excess weight was lost over three years. The procedure was complicated by dental caries and problems with the temporomandibular joint, where the jaw articulates with the skull. A significant number of patients could not tolerate the procedure and insisted upon having the caps removed.

All patients regained most of the weight lost after the wires were removed. In a number of patients, the jaws were rewired. And this was accompanied by further weight loss. This again was regained after the wires had been removed.

In some of the studies, a nylon thread was placed around the central abdomen. And as waste measurements increased, so did the tightness of the thread. This, in turn, produced discomfort for the patient: the thread cut into the tissues and created an additional stimulus to eat less.

THE INTRAGASTRIC BALLOON

A device that was used over 20 years ago was the intragastric balloon. The rationale behind this was that the presence of a balloon in the stomach would create a feeling of early satiety. The balloon would restrict the amount of space available for food taken at meals. The stomach has the capacity to accommodate about 1 1/2 L of fluid. It undergoes a process known as adaptive relaxation.

This process enables us to eat or drink large amounts without feeling excessively full. This adaptive relaxation is a method of muscular relaxation which increases the volume of the stomach from about 50mL in the resting state, to 1 1/2 L in its fully distended state. Beyond full distention, a feeling of discomfort arises. And any further distention, beyond that point, will cause vomiting.

Approximately 20 years ago, the author introduced the Taylor intragastric balloon, which was published in the *American Journal of Gastroenterology*. This was a silicone, free-floating balloon, which encompassed the concept. The Taylor balloon, constructed from high-grade medical silicone, had a capacity of about 600mL. This balloon, when deflated, was packed into the end of a tube or introducer. The tube was inserted into the stomach. And through an inner tube, the balloon was filled with fluid. A small amount of radio-opaque material was introduced into the balloon so that it could be seen under X-ray.

Fluid was introduced into the balloon, and it expanded and came out of the tube that was used for introduction. When 600mL of fluid was inserted, the inner tube used for inflation was removed from the valve in the wall of the balloon. And then, the balloon was left free-floating in the stomach. This balloon created the feeling of early satiety. And weight loss was recorded over a two-to-three-month period. However, after this time, no further weight loss was recorded and, in some patients, weight was regained.

On reflection, even the Taylor balloon was probably too small. The concept of an intragastric balloon as a method of treating obesity is not altogether inappropriate. In light of the stomach's ability to expand to a volume of about 1 1/2 L, it would appear that the early research done in this field employed balloons that were of an inadequate volume to achieve the desired result. It is conceivable that if a balloon with a volume in excess of 1 1/2L were used, the results would improve.

New materials are now available that are extremely thin-walled and capable of marked expansion within the stomach. The material is inert and is not likely to cause problems within the stomach. If an adequate amount of space is taken up in the stomach, then the ability to eat around the balloon would become increasingly difficult. And therefore, weight would be lost in the same way as it decreases with gastric restrictive surgical procedures, which we will discuss. It is conceivable that a self-inflating pill could be devised. This pill, when swallowed, spontaneously expands to the required volume in the stomach so as to restrict the intake of large amounts of food.

GASTROPLASTY

Gastric restrictive procedures are designed to limit the intake of food by creating a small gastric pouch. This is a method through which the stomach is partitioned using staples to create a small upper pouch. This pouch empties slowly, either into the lower normal stomach or into a loop of the small intestine. This is then joined to the small pouch.

Gastric restrictive procedures were introduced by Dr. Mason of Iowa in the early 1970s. When they evolved, it became apparent that the size of the small gastric pouch could only be something along the lines of 20 to 30mL. This resulted in gastric pouch distention after eating only a very small amount of food. And the feeling of fullness stopped the patient from further eating. Should the patient continue to eat under these circumstances, vomiting would occur.

When gastroplasty alone is performed, it does not bypass any part of the intestinal tract. This small pouch of the stomach empties through a very small opening. It is done so that the rate of gastric emptying of food into the lower stomach or intestine is slow. And therefore, the feeling of satiety persists for some time. The physical restriction of eating caused by gastroplasty requires patients to ingest three to six small meals per day.

Patients are encouraged to eat solid food and to sip high-calorie drinks or eat ice cream. By doing this, they can, to some extent, overcome the effects of the gastroplasty. People who drink high-calorie liquids in association with gastroplasty are also prone to develop "dumping," a sensation of nausea, dizziness, and abdominal discomfort.

One of the problems with early gastroplasty was that the gastric outlet tended to stretch with time. This allowed more rapid gastric emptying than was optimal. To overcome this, the gastric outlet was frequently banded by using synthetic materials such as Dacron, Marlex, or silicone.

VERTICAL-BANDED OR RING GASTROPLASTY

Gastroplasties interfere with the physiology of eating to a lesser extent than jejunoileal bypass procedures. Their evolution over recent years culminated in the development of two major types of open procedure: the vertical-banded gastroplasty and the Silastic ring, vertical gastroplasty.

In the vertical-banded gastroplasty, four layers of staples are placed parallel to the lesser curvature of the stomach. And in the outlet of the gastroplasty, a hole is punched through the stomach to create a new outlet. This outlet is reinforced by a band five to 5.5cm in length. This prevents the outlet from stretching. The total volume of the gastroplasty is of the order of 20mL.

The Silastic ring vertical gastroplasty is performed by placing four layers of staples parallel to the lesser curvature of the stomach and placing a Silastic ring around these at the gastric outlet, thus creating a new small gastric outlet that would restrict the rate of emptying of the stomach. This operation is performed by a specially designed notched staple gun. The results of vertical banded gastroplasty and Silastic ring vertical gastroplasty are virtually the same and depend essentially upon the size of the gastric outlet and the volume of the gastric pouch.

The reason for introducing gastroplasty was that it was felt it would produce fewer acute complications than intestinal bypass. Vertical banded gastroplasty might have appeared safer and a less complicated procedure than gastroplasty with bypass or intestinal bypass. Yet, several studies comparing the two techniques showed very little difference in outcome.

With gastric bypass, gastroplasty, and jejunoileal bypass, there is always a risk of leakage at the sites where the bowel is joined together with staples. And such leakage can be difficult to detect in the post-operative period. The patient's morbidly obese state makes examination of the abdomen difficult in the early post-op. And obesity also tends to delay the clinical manifestations of septic complications. This might occur until these have reached an advanced stage. In this case, they can become irreversible and go on to lead to multiple organ failure. This carries a high mortality.

A problem commonly associated with obesity is gastroesophageal reflux disease (GERD). This condition is virtually cured by the performance of gastroplasty. The small gastric pouch is incapable of generating enough acid to cause significant damage at the lower end of the esophagus.

Moreover, it prevents bile from refluxing from the duodenum through the stomach into the esophagus. GERD is better prevented by gastric bypass than by vertical banded gastroplasty. However, the latter procedure is also successful in ameliorating the symptoms of most patients who have obesity and GERD. The major advantage of vertical banded gastroplasty over gastric bypass is that it is easier to perform. Furthermore, it is not associated with vitamin and iron deficiency or with the dumping syndrome.

In dumping syndrome, the patient primarily experiences a sensation of lightheadedness and nausea. This is due to rapid early emptying of the stomach. All forms of gastroplasty result in the retention of solid food, sometimes leading to gastric outlet obstruction. This condition may require endoscopy and the clearance of the obstructing food debris.

Studies that compared gastric bypass with vertical banded gastroplasty seem to show a greater weight loss with the former procedure. Weight loss after vertical banded gastroplasty was, on the whole, something of the order of 60% of excess body weight at two years and 40% at three years.

After a gastric bypass procedure, patients lost between 65% of their excess body weight at two years and about 60% at three years. After this certain amount of time, there was a tendency for these groups of patients to begin to regain weight. The weight gain may be due to stretching of the pouch with the resulting increased volume of the gastric reservoir, widening of the gastric outlet. Or alternatively, erosion of staples along the line of the gastroplasty.

GASTRIC BANDING

In the late 1980s, the concept of placing a band of inflexible material around the upper stomach was introduced. Surgeons initially used a band of silicone tubing or polypropylene mesh to reinforce the outlet, creating approximately a 50mL volume of gastric pouch. The band was in operation, tied around a "bougie" or tube placed in the stomach to control the size of the gastric outlet. The advantage of these procedures was the simplicity. And the lack of any anastomosis might ultimately break down, leak, and give rise to serious complications.

THE LAP-BAND

Several groups of surgeons used non-adjustable gastric banding for a number of years, and this led to a significant incidence of gastric outlet obstruction. An attempt to overcome the problem was made by introducing an adjustable gastric band. The principle of this procedure involved the use of a balloon in relation to the gastric band. This could be adjusted in its volume so as to alter the size of the outlet of the gastric pouch.

The adjustable gastric band was available in Europe for some years before it gained popularity in the United States. A major reason for its popularity is the relative simplicity of the insertion of the balloon. And of course, the reduction in complications associated with the procedure.

A further advantage was that the procedure could be performed laparoscopically. This led to a shorter hospital stay and more rapid postoperative recovery. Trials in the United States were initiated with the adjustable gastric band. This was approved by the FDA as an obesity treatment in June 2000 based on a pre-market approval application that contained data from a trial of more than 290 morbidly obese Americans. In addition to this, international data was collected in Australia, Europe, and Mexico. This trial demonstrated that more than 70% of these patients who were followed for three years lost and maintained an average of more than 18% of their excess body weight.

This weight loss represented some 40% of their excess body weight. This, in many ways, was not too impressive. Moreover, increasing experience with the lap-band tended to produce somewhat inferior results. The band, however, was not without complications. Early in the placement experience, almost 20% of bands migrated. Either the pouch or the esophagus dilated in the first year after placement due to migration of the band, leading to failure of the weight-reducing procedure.

The basic techniques for successfully placing an adjustable gastric band rely upon the creation of a suitably sized pouch close to the junction of the esophagus and the upper stomach. Then, minimal trauma along the stomach while tunneling behind it. Avoiding damage to the band while placing it around the stomach. And finally, creating a tension-free band that is uniformly placed around the upper stomach.

Band slippage has been a problem. And the best way to avoid this was for the surgeon to be extremely precise: to the point that the site he chose to place the band around the stomach was appropriate. The band should encircle an area of the stomach that is less than 20mL in volume, this being the gastric pouch. Finally, the lower stomach is folded over the band to create a loose tunnel. This can be done by placing a few sutures in the stomach wall and across the pouch.

An additional advantage of the adjustable band is that it is relatively simple to reverse. Although clearly, reversal for patients who have undergone weight loss surgery results in a return to the pre-operative weight, despite the patient trying to convince the surgeon that this will not be the case. Plus, removing the band is often a complicated procedure due to the dense adhesions that form between the gastric wall and the band itself.

Techniques were introduced to modify the device and reduce the complications of use. However, the overall results were far from satisfactory. And also, the use of the band has now largely been abandoned and replaced, chiefly by the gastric sleeve procedure. A further problem was the erosion of the band through the stomach wall and into the gastric cavity.

GASTRIC BYPASS: THE ROUX-EN-Y TECHNIQUE

When gastric bypass was first introduced, weight loss was variable, and patients complained of bile vomiting and reflux disease due to bile washing back into the stomach and esophagus. This led to the development of the Roux-en-Y gastroplasty.

In this procedure, the gastric pouch must be small: 10 to 30 milliliters. The outlet of the pouch should be about 1 cm in diameter. Bile should be diverted to a point lower down the intestinal tract. And the loop of the small bowel created to drain the gastric pouch should be a minimum of 60 cm in length. This is before it is joined by the point at which the bile enters the rest of the intestine. Out of these factors, probably the most important are the presence of a small gastric pouch and the diversion of bile in a fashion described as the Roux-en-Y technique. This concept was described by the Swiss surgeon Roux in the early 20th century.

The Roux loop not only prevents bile from entering the stomach and thereby causing vomiting and pain, but also, for some reason—still not fully understood—causes a reduction in appetite and slows gastric emptying.

Thus, the combination of a small gastric pouch and a Roux-en-Y anastomosis has turned out to be the most efficacious way of achieving acceptable amounts of sustained weight loss in morbidly obese patients. Therefore, this operation should be regarded as the "gold standard" against which other operations must be compared.

Results, in terms of weight loss, are superior to those that can be achieved by the adjustable gastric band. In stark contrast to the band, however, this is a major operative procedure as it involves the creation of several anastomoses. These are areas where the bowel has to be divided and joined together. Wherever an anastomosis occurs, there is a potential for leakage, and leakage is potentially fatal.

Over the past 20 years, the sophistication of procedures that can be performed laparoscopically has increased dramatically, and it is now possible to perform a Roux-en-Y Gastric Bypass with low morbidity and mortality. However, the risk of this procedure in the morbidly obese patient should never be underestimated.

Overall, a significant number of complications and deaths have been recorded. And this has led the American Society of Bariatric Surgeons to look most carefully at both those who perform these procedures and where they are carried out.

Clearly, there is something to be said for the development of a specialized "bariatric center" where surgeons devote themselves entirely to the performance of bariatric surgery: on the grounds that "the more procedures one does, the better one becomes." This would appear to be a significant and powerful argument in favor of the creation of such centers and the development of a specialty of bariatric surgery.

INDICATIONS FOR THE ROUX-EN-Y GASTRIC BYPASS

The indications for gastric bypass are:

1. The patient should have a body mass index greater than or equal to 40 or a body mass index in excess of 35 in a patient who has comorbidities. For example, conditions like sleep apnea or diabetes.
2. The patient should be willing to undergo a period of long-term follow-up and comply with medical treatment so as to avoid potential nutritional side effects.
3. The patient must be capable of understanding the nature of the procedure that is being performed and its potential consequences. And thus should be well enough informed to give meaningful consent.
4. There must be no history of alcohol or substance abuse.
5. The presence of any major psychiatric disorder, especially depression associated with suicidal ideations, is a contraindication.

Other contraindications include serious medical conditions that increase the risk of surgery, lack of family support, and failure to understand the constraints placed upon the patient who has undergone this form of surgery.

OUTCOMES

The procedure of Roux-en-Y Gastric Bypass can vary considerably from surgeon to surgeon; for example, it may be done as an open operation or performed laparoscopically. The sizes of the gastric pouches vary, and this is crucial. The length of the roux loop can also differ and create varying results. The addition or absence of some form of gastric ring outlets or constraint device can also vary the outcome. The method of carrying out anastomoses of the bowel can vary between stapling and hand-sewn techniques. This variation also happens with the length and nature of the intestinal loops. And also, where they are placed in relation to the colon may also vary.

Many versions of this procedure have been described; probably the most reliable is that which creates a 20 to 30mL stapled gastric pouch, a 1 cm diameter gastroenter-ostomy, which is handsewn, and a 40 to 60 cm Roux loop. This is major surgery! And when carried out in the morbidly obese patient, the risks of anesthesia and surgery are considerably higher than for similar procedures carried out in those who are of normal weight.

There is the risk of *perioperative mortality* with this procedure. This is the order of 1%, in the best of hands. The most common cause of death is sepsis. This leakage occurs at the joining of the bowel. Other causes of mortality are myocardial infarction and pulmonary embolism. Respiratory failure can also occur, particularly in the super obese.

RESULTS

People have received exceptional results in terms of weight control from this procedure. From the mean preoperative weight of 300 pounds, the average weight after one year is of the order of 190 pounds. After one year, the weight usually stabilizes below this level. However, very few achieve the ideal range of weight. The loss of 100 pounds or more is very significant to their lifestyle and their associated medical problems.

Most of the patients undergoing this form of surgery are female, and the mortality in males tends to be higher.

In addition, the results are not quite as good in males as in females. Patients over the age of 55 have about a threefold increased mortality rate associated with the surgery.

Following laparoscopic gastric bypass, the results in terms of weight loss are similar to those achieved with the open operation. However, the recovery with the laparoscopic procedure is usually much quicker. It must be realized, however, that any procedure performed laparoscopically involves an added difficulty when compared with performing it by the open route. The main reasons for mortality following the laparoscopic approach have, again, been due principally to leakage of the bowel at the anastomosis.

By and large, laparoscopic surgery is associated with a longer operative time. However, there is less blood loss, with a much shorter hospital stay and a faster convalescence. The weight loss at one year is comparable between the open and laparoscopically performed procedures. A major advantage of the laparoscopic approach is that there are fewer wound problems thereafter, in particular, no risk of an incisional hernia.

LONG-TERM ADVANTAGES

Following surgery, full remission of Type 2 diabetes, sleep apnea, hypertension, infertility, fatty infiltration of the liver, gastroesophageal reflux, and arthritis may be expected to occur. It is unlikely that in the future the mortality rate will be significantly lessened from its already low level. It is of great importance that the patient undergoing this form of surgery must understand the risks associated with it.

The risks of the conditions associated with morbid obesity, however, in the long term, are much greater than those associated with the surgery. And these risks are certainly minimized after the surgery. Therefore, surgery not only greatly reduces overall risk but also the cost of the medical treatment as well.

BILIOPANCREATIC DIVERSION

As food passes from the stomach into the duodenum, it comes into contact with bile and pancreatic juice. These fluids are essential for the normal digestive process. Pancreatic juice, in particular, contains the powerful enzymes amylase, lipase, and trypsin. These chemicals break down large molecules of carbohydrate, fat, and protein, respectively, into much smaller molecules suitable for absorption in the intestine. It is these enzymes that digest the pieces of steak you eat for dinner.

In addition, bile is necessary for fat absorption, and limiting its contact with food decreases fat absorption. When bile is diverted much lower down the intestine, this leads to a much shorter length of intestine through which the food may be absorbed. As a result, it significantly limits it. If the bile is placed low down the intestine, then some degree of malabsorption will occur.

In other words, not all of the food products are completely absorbed. Some are lost from the intestinal tract. In this way, some of the calories that are ingested are not utilized, saving them from contributing to the overall calorie intake and the obese state. The principle underlying the more radical biliopancreatic diversion operation is to insert the bile lower down the intestine so that a degree of malabsorption occurs. This procedure is combined with a gastroplasty and is used for the super obese patient, producing much increased and radical amounts of weight loss. There is a risk of malabsorption and vitamin and mineral depletion. As a result, long-term follow-up and careful observation for these complications are necessary. There are two varieties of this procedure that are performed: the Scopinaro operation and the Duodenal Switch procedure. These form a functional and ultimate outcome effect that is very similar.

THE GASTRIC SLEEVE PROCEDURE

The game changer in weight-reducing surgery for the average patient occurred about 25 years ago. Gastric sleeve resection is an operation that drastically reduces the capacity of the stomach but retains its nerve supply. It does this through the vagus nerve and preserves the normal control of gastric emptying into the duodenum through the pylorus. The rest of the gastrointestinal tract remains intact and unchanged, acting physiologically. So, there is little absorptive change or challenge. The underlying strategy goes back to reducing the capacity of the stomach. But in a somewhat different way than with the earlier operations described earlier.

Gastric sleeve resection creates a small, narrow tube of stomach extending from the inlet at the esophagus to the outlet through the normal pylorus. In creating this narrow tube of stomach, the greater volume and capacity of the stomach are removed, leaving a narrow sleeve with all of its original nerve supply intact. This relates to its functional capacity. The procedure is performed laparoscopically, dividing the full thickness of the stomach along its whole length parallel to the lesser curvature. The divided lateral and remaining volume of the stomach—having been disconnected from the newly created sleeve—is then completely removed from the abdomen through a small incision.

The procedure is simpler, safer to perform, and effective. The surgery is performed as a day-case procedure, and recovery is typically fast. Though less radical than the Roux-en-Y Gastric Bypass, the weight loss is usually good and well sustained. However, in most cases, less weight will be lost than that achieved with the more radical Roux-en-Y Gastric Bypass. The procedure has become probably the most widely performed operation for weight loss and is a very safe and effective one.

Its role is probably optimized as lying somewhat below the Roux-en-Y Gastric Bypass, but safer, simpler, and more physiological. And it is ideal for those in the middle of the overweight range. It has been shown to be effective in improving the complications of obesity, including diabetes. Good long-term results have been reported with few side effects. And the operation has become the most popular one performed overall.

CHAPTER 19: COMPLICATIONS OF BARIATRIC SURGERY

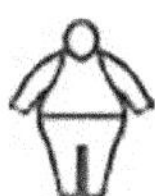

The vast increase in obesity is undoubtedly going to herald increased mortality in the untreated obese population for some time to come, and it is increasing. This is already becoming manifest in health-related problems such as diabetes, coronary artery disease, and hypertension. It has been shown that the cost of treating patients for the comorbidities of the morbidly obese state is greater than the cost associated with surgery for their obesity. However, surgery is complex, and there are risks.

The morbidly obese patient presents special challenges to the surgeon and anesthesiologist in the healthcare team. Venous access is more difficult. Intubation for anesthesia is complex, and airway management can be a problem. Handling and mobilization of the patient involves many staff and is often difficult. Overall, special and more intensive care is required for the obese undergoing abdominal surgery than for those of normal weight.

As stated previously, the mortality associated with obesity surgery is of the order of 1%. There is a mortality associated with all operative procedures. The definition of a postoperative mortality is a death that occurs within 30 days of the operation. Clearly, within 30 days of the operation, some patients are going to develop heart attacks and others life-threatening problems irrespective of the surgery. But equally, problems from the surgery can accrue, and these can be life-threatening.

During the postoperative period, breathing is more difficult, and ambulation is often slow. This leads to chest infection, collapse of the lung bases, and the formation of clots of blood in the lower limbs, venous thrombosis. The risk associated with thrombosis in the deep veins of the lower limbs is that of pulmonary embolism.

Pulmonary embolism occurs when a thrombus or clot, usually in the lower limbs, becomes detached and floats through the circulation to block the main arterial output from the heart to the lungs. Fatal pulmonary embolus is more likely to occur in obese patients than in normal-weight patients, despite the use of low-dose anticoagulant drugs. This may lower the likelihood of this life-threatening complication. In patients who have arteriosclerosis, surgery presents a major stressful incident. This increases the risk of coronary artery thrombosis and death associated with it.

A major risk associated with weight reduction surgery is leakage from the suture lines where the bowel has been joined together either by direct suturing or by stapling. Surgeons routinely test suture lines at the time of operation. But unfortunately, post-operative leaks occur in a minority of patients and can lead to the development of peritonitis and death.

Leakage can occur from any point at which the intestine is either stapled or joined to another piece of gut. These leaks may be difficult to detect clinically in a timely fashion in view of the obese state of the patient's abdomen. At the first clinical suspicion, the patient must be thoroughly investigated. And if a leak is identified, further surgery is mandatory. A later complication can occur at sites where the intestine is joined, resulting in the formation of a stricture. A "stricture" is a narrowing of the bowel that leads to partial or complete obstruction. In association with strictures, ulceration may occur. And that may, in turn, lead to gastrointestinal bleeding.

Another potential problem associated with major gastric bypass procedures is internal hernia. In this condition, there is an abnormal protrusion of the loop of intestine through a defect inside the abdomen. Such an abnormal protrusion can lead to either intestinal obstruction. Or in the worst-case scenario, strangulation of the gut with peritonitis.

More intensive surgery is mandatory to correct this. Morbidly obese patients have an increased likelihood of gallstone formation. This propensity is further increased postoperatively. Some surgeons routinely remove the gallbladder at the time of performing obesity surgery. But this, of course, creates a further potential for postoperative problems, so it is by no means a universal practice.

Rapid weight loss in itself increases the incidence of gallstone formation. This can give rise to serious complications like jaundice and pancreatitis. The most common complication following open obesity surgery is wound infection. This may lead either to a breakdown of the wound or to the development of an incisional hernia. The presence of large amounts of fat on the abdominal wall predisposes the patient to the development of wound infections. And unfortunately, when these occur, they may become complex: abscesses may form, and the wound may need to be reopened and packed.

All of these complications delay recovery after the procedure. This separation of the abdominal muscle occurs either as a result of infection or breakdown of the wound. The wound may require resuture, or at best, a ventral hernia may develop. This will ultimately need to be repaired. Repair of these incisional hernias in the obese patient can in itself be a complex procedure. This often necessitates reconstruction of the wound by applying sheets of mesh to reinforce the reconstructed wound.

One of the major advantages of laparoscopic approaches is that wound problems rarely occur. There are several small "port sites." This occasionally gives rise to either infections or postoperative bowel obstruction.

Laparoscopic surgery, however, adds another layer of complexity to the procedure. Pouch size and loop length are more difficult to assess. At the same time, precise stitching is more difficult to perform using the laparoscopic approach.

Following gastric surgery, the control of gastric emptying is impaired, and dumping can occur. Dumping is a condition characterized by sweating, nausea, weakness, palpitations, lightheadedness, and vomiting. It is due to a combination of fluid loss and hypoglycemia, mainly due to rapid gastric emptying.

The use of the gastric band is associated with specific complications, perhaps the most serious of which is displacement of the band. This placement of the band is associated with slipping or prolapse of the stomach through the band. And this can give rise to obstruction and the necessity for further surgery.

Nausea, vomiting, and reflux disease are also associated with the use of the band. These problems can, to some extent, be corrected by altering the degree of inflation of the adjustable band. Yet, sometimes further surgery or endoscopic stretching of the outlet of the gastric pouch may be required. An occasional complication of the band has been erosion through the wall of the stomach. This is clearly a serious complication.

The older malabsorption procedures, such as jejunoileal bypass, were abandoned because of severe side effects. The major of these was fatty infiltration of the liver. This could lead to cirrhosis and liver failure, together with electrolyte problems. Electrolyte derangements can be life-threatening; in particular, a fall in serum potassium can give rise to abnormalities of cardiac function, sometimes resulting in sudden cardiac arrest.

Only a small number of patients develop these life-threatening complications. But it could not be predicted who was most vulnerable. And therefore, these procedures ultimately were abandoned, even though some good long-term results were obtained.

In the long term, it is important that patients adhere to dietary recommendations, in particular taking vitamin and mineral supplements. Without these, patients are prone to establish vitamin or mineral deficiencies such as Wernicke's encephalopathy, scurvy, and vitamin B12 deficiency. They also include mineral deficiencies such as calcium, zinc, and magnesium. Females who are menstruating must take an iron supplement to avoid the development of anemia.

CHAPTER 20: LONG-TERM MORBIDITY AND MORTALITY IN MORBIDLY OBESE PATIENTS

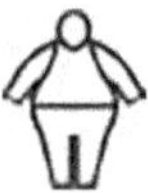

After smoking, obesity is the second leading cause of preventable premature death in the United States. It is estimated that there are 500,000 deaths attributable to obesity in the United States each year.

The epidemic of obesity is not confined to the United States and affects most Westernized countries. The related comorbidities discussed earlier in this text lead to physical and psychological problems, together with premature death.

Bariatric surgery undoubtedly produces large amounts of weight loss in cooperative patients. But until recently, little has been known about the comparisons of long-term morbidity in those who have undergone obesity surgery. Up until the modern days, there has not been a population-based study demonstrating a significant impact of surgically induced weight loss on mortality and the potential for comorbidity.

A study from Canada has addressed these problems, testing the hypothesis that weight-reducing surgery reduces long-term mortality and morbidity in morbidly obese patients. This study from McGill University Health Center compared the morbidity and mortality of a cohort of morbidly obese patients treated with bariatric surgery with morbidly obese controls who had not been treated surgically. This is a large study containing a total of 1,119 patients who underwent bariatric surgery for the treatment of morbid obesity between 1986 and 2002.

A maximum of six controls were identified for each bariatric subject. The single-payer healthcare system in Canada enables health expenditures and clinical outcomes to be documented for all citizens. And this greatly aids in the feasibility of conducting research studies of this nature. A total of 5,746 controls were included in this study.

The surgical procedure used for the morbidly obese patient was Roux-en-Y Gastric Bypass. The costs of healthcare were determined by searching the national health database over a five-year period. Patients treated surgically lost a mean of 67% of their initial weight.

In comparison with controls, bariatric surgery patients had significantly lower incidence rates for the following clinical conditions: cancer, cardiovascular and circulatory problems, diabetes mellitus, endocrinological problems, genitourinary problems, infectious diseases, musculoskeletal problems, diseases of the nervous system, psychiatric and mental disease, respiratory problems, and dermatological disorders.

There was a fourfold reduction in cancer, a fivefold reduction in cardiovascular and circulatory problems, and a reduction in respiratory disorders in the surgically treated group. During the period of study, the mortality in the surgically treated group was reduced by 90% in comparison to the control group. The mortality in the surgical group included perioperative deaths, which had an incidence of 0.4%.

Another way to describe the mortality data is a relative reduction of mortality of 18.9% by surgery that produced a sustained 67% excess weight loss compared with controls who did not undergo surgery. During the period of study, the total in-hospital days were significantly lower in the bariatric surgery patients when compared with controls.

Also, bariatric surgery patients made fewer physician visits in the five-year follow-up group, including the planned yearly follow-up surgery group. Bariatric surgery patients had 50% fewer hospitalizations and significantly reduced hospitalization rates for cancers, cardiovascular, and circulatory conditions. This included conditions like hypertension, infections, and other major conditions.

In the bariatric cohort had significantly reduced rates of hospitalization for digestive conditions when compared with surgical patients. Typically, on average, the total direct healthcare costs for the control group were 45% higher compared with bariatric surgically treated patients. The finding of significantly reduced healthcare use rates and total direct healthcare costs is imperative from a societal and health economic point of view. Why? This is the case because healthcare services and costs associated with surgery were included in the total cost for the bariatric surgery group. The total benefit for the surgically treated patient would be greater than 45% if indirect costs were included.

This is an excellent study that has great strengths, particularly relating to the selection of the cohorts. Matching of the cases and controls with respect to age, gender, and duration of disease reduces the possibility of confounding from these factors. This is mainly because both are potentially associated with morbidity indices studied and with increased risk for mortality.

Furthermore, the random selection of controls from an administrative database reduces selection bias and bias by indication that would have been introduced if hospital-based controls were used. This study has produced emphatic evidence supporting the implementation of bariatric surgery in the management of the morbidly obese patient. It is a direct pointer to the healthcare industry. It indicates the implementation of bariatric surgery and the encouragement of the appropriate patient to undergo that surgery. It is beneficial not only in terms of morbidity and mortality but also in healthcare economics.

It will now be of great interest to see what the impact of the new weight-reducing drugs like Wegovy has on the long-term effects of weight loss and the complications of obesity. Because, in recent studies, these drugs have been shown to produce large amounts of weight loss. And they also appear to be effective in reducing heart attacks, strokes, diabetes, and vascular disease. These drugs are expensive. However, in the long term, the overall equation could work in their favor. They could have a major effect on the number of cases undergoing surgical treatment for obesity.

CHAPTER 21: SUPERMARKETS: THE FOOD WE BUY

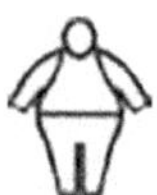

Foods bought from supermarkets can be of questionable value. For example, more fat is found in three slices of bread than in a calorie-rich Mars bar. Some breakfast cereals contain more than 15% fat, and some best-selling ready-made meals have more than triple the fat of other similar products. The amount of fat in pizzas can vary from 15% to 4%.

Supermarkets often provide unchallenging comfort cuisine, rows and rows of ready-made foods from chicken pot pies to sponge cakes that once would have been made at home. These products contain palm oil emulsifiers, hydrogenated vegetable oil, and a bewildering array of additives. These are used partly to ensure that foods last longer, taste better, and cost less. Fat is abundant, cheap, and can prolong the shelf life of products, adding an attractive texture and taste. The result, over the past few decades, has been rising fat content in most popular foods purchased.

Product longevity is a further issue. For example, a homemade lemon cake containing 10% fat would be stale and inedible after two or three days. All the while, a supermarket cake with 20% fat tastes the same in three months as it does now.

Fat emulsifiers are based on the chemistry that came out of the soap industry. They make fat more palatable.

The result is that some breads contain 12% fat, whereas, in contrast, full-fat milk contains only 4% fat.

According to the Atkins philosophy, this might not seem to be so important. But in all probability, it is extremely so. The reason is that trans fatty acids from hydrogenated vegetable fat used in cakes, cookies, and margarine are in themselves a health risk.

Trans fatty acids cannot be properly digested. And the body simply stores them as fat. There is evidence that trans fatty acids are involved in the formation of cholesterol deposits in the blood vessels in diabetes and in obesity. On the other hand, monounsaturated fats such as those found in avocados and nuts are believed to be beneficial. This is especially when taken in moderation, possibly protecting against heart disease.

It may be, therefore, that not all of the obesity revolution is the responsibility of the consumer. But it is contributed to, in some significant degree, by supermarkets which control about 90% of food consumption. Supermarkets are making some progress in providing healthy alternatives, and labeling of energy content in food is becoming increasingly detailed and helpful.

In the United Kingdom, a House of Commons select committee has recently criticized the food industry for not doing enough to promote healthy foods. They are introducing a traffic light system policy for labeling foods: those with increasing calorie intake are in the red zone.

A study compiled by 126 nutrition professionals with the American Diabetes Association—including sport nutritionists, cookbook and nutrition book authors, heads of hospital wellness programs, and university weight researchers—agreed that we cannot afford to allow the overweight population to increase over the next 20 years. The reasoning is that it has been over the last equivalent.

It was emphasized that a strategy must be formulated to prevent the one to two pounds that the average American gains each year from continuing.

About 65% of adults in the United States now weigh too much. This study determined the following major obstacles:

1) Most people do not have a realistic idea of portion sizes. Restaurants often contribute to the problem, that are at least twice the recommended serving size
2) Children don't change bad eating habits for good; instead, they choose fad diets which they adhere to, in the short term only. And then revert to their previous eating habits
3) Most people consider exercise a drudgery and rarely stay with exercise programs.
4) There is a large reluctance to change eating habits as people become "addicted" to their favorite foods.
5) People fail to realize that there is no such thing as a miracle diet.

What the overweight want to hear is that losing weight is quick, easy, miraculous, and involves little effort. No such system exists! The nutritionists in this study felt that a big problem was that activity had been squeezed out of people's lives by modern technology.

Moving from cars, to desks, to television screens, and to computers has ruled exercise out of most people's way of existence. However, exercise is of fundamental importance not only from the point of view of obesity but also from that of keeping healthy.

CHAPTER 22: VISITING THE SUPERMARKET: WHAT TO PURCHASE?

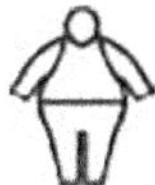

Wherever we go today, we are faced with a plethora of food items that are on sale. Even at the gas station, quite a large array of foods is available, chiefly fast foods and those that are high in carbohydrate and fat content. These are also relatively inexpensive.

Clearly, buying and taking into the house the wrong type of food is a fundamental problem in the obesity equation. And if bad food is not available in the house, then it is not going to be eaten during periods of vulnerability. It is important, therefore, in carrying out grocery shopping, that healthy foods are purchased. And those that are harmful to health or have a particularly high glycemic index should be avoided.

When visiting the supermarket, go easy on breads, rice, cereals, and pasta. There is no need to eat breakfast cereals, and very little need to eat bread. Pasta is also something that can readily be avoided. When bread is purchased, it should be the wholemeal or the whole wheat variety. In the end, white sliced bread should be avoided.

Pizzas should be avoided, as should cakes, bagels, and cookies. There is no need to have refined granulated sugar in the house. When entering the supermarket, you are usually faced with an array of the foregoing foodstuffs.

Resist the temptation to buy them and move on to the fruits and vegetables section.

Here, not only are the glycemic indexes lower and the number of calories taken less, but also these foods contain essential vitamins and minerals. They are imperative for good health.

Whenever visiting the food section of the store, go for green colored items such as lettuce, broccoli, asparagus, and spinach. Vegetables are better than fruits, and fruits that are somewhat undesirable are bananas and melons. The only fruit or vegetable that contains a significant amount of fat is the avocado. However, this is healthy fat and is good to eat. There is also some fat in coconuts.

Ultimate timesaving purchases can be prepared, such as salads. They are readily available and do not involve any cooking. Roots that are dark red, purple, or black are often healthy to eat. However, jams and jellies like blueberry jellies often have a considerable amount of added sugar.

Along the dairy aisle, low-fat dairy products are an excellent source of food and nutrition and contain crucial minerals such as calcium. These minerals are crucial, particularly in women, to prevent metabolic bone disease such as osteoporosis. Buy either skim or 1% low-fat milk.

Fat-free milk may be fortified with additional protein. And along with fat, it contains more calcium. Low-fat cottage cheese, sour cream, and yogurt are quite healthy. Also, low-fat cheese is a reasonable addition to the diet. One of the best cheeses along these lines is mozzarella.

Sugar-filled dressings like ranch should be avoided. However, they are now being produced with significantly less sugar content, and honey mustard is also available for purchase. These items contain no sugar at all and taste very much like the traditional product. Buttermilk garlic, as a whole, contains little fat. Eggs are a useful source of protein. And despite the cholesterol content of the yolk, they are not a bad form of nutrition. The average egg only contains 60 calories.

When entering the meat area, concentrate on lean white meat. Turkey and chicken slices can contain less than 2% fat. Or even in the case of turkey, no fat at all. Steak, in particular sirloin and tenderloin, can be eaten once or twice a week. However, the fat on the outside should be removed.

Even pork is healthy to eat, provided the fat is taken off. In the poultry section, white poultry is lower in fat than dark. The skin of turkeys, chickens, and ducks is high in fat and calories and should be removed.

Seafood is excellent, particularly white fish. Great emphasis has been placed on eating salmon. It always had a great reputation. This has, however, been somewhat tarnished by adverse publicity relating to carcinogens that are present in farm-raised salmon. There is some dispute regarding the authenticity of these claims. And although these carcinogens probably exist, they are most likely present only in minute quantities. And thus unlikely to affect health adversely.

Tofu is an excellent source of both protein and calcium. Nuts can be bought because they are possibly helpful in preventing cardiovascular disease. You will need to buy some butter or margarine, and it probably does not matter which. However, the module reading must not contain too many trans fatty acids.

Purchase low-or no-calorie sweeteners such as Splenda. Adverse publicity about saccharin, which is high in products such as Sweet'n Low, has been continuously raised. However, it may just be an exaggeration. Almost everyone tolerates sweeteners well. One sweetener, aspartame, has now been withdrawn from the market because of anxieties relating to carcinogenesis. Whatever the downside of eating sweeteners, these are very much less than those associated with ingesting large amounts of sugar.

It is important, therefore, when visiting the supermarket to employ the right strategy. Why? Because what you walk out with is certainly what you're going to eat. This probably gives as good a reflection as anything regarding your food intake and how it relates to your health and weight.

CHAPTER 23: OBESITY—WHAT SHOULD I DO?

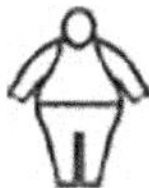

This book provides an overview of the major aspects of obesity. Specific advice needs to be tailored to the individual. However, broad general categories have been outlined that can be separated from the therapeutic point of view.

Therapy is not only instrumental in treating obesity but also absolutely effective in the management of its complications. Treatment can be divided into calorie restriction, diet, exercise, behavioral therapy, drug therapy, and surgery.

All are disciplines and strategies that may have to be adopted to cope with the problem in the long term. Compromise is essential in all aspects of life. And we must remember that compromise begins with a trip to the supermarket. If it is not in the refrigerator, you're less likely to be tempted by it. The bottom line in achieving weight loss is that the patient must take in fewer calories than the calories that are expended. All diets depend on this fundamental principle.

Food needs to be rationed to some extent; there are no hard and fast rules about the way this should be done, but restriction in some form is essential. The Atkins diet, which originally produced massive amounts of weight loss, was the major introduction to the importance of avoiding carbohydrates. It probably went too far in stating that if you avoid carbohydrates, you can eat what you want. This is not the case. And therefore, the South Beach and the Sugar Busters diets are superior.

Given that the initial premise of avoiding carbohydrates can be adhered to, then caloric restriction is easier than any carbohydrate-containing diet. This is because large volumes of food comprising only protein and fat are difficult to eat without carbohydrates.

Present yourself with a huge plate of sliced chicken breast, no sauces and no additives, and you will rapidly tire of eating it. It will be difficult to consume. Perhaps bacon and eggs are more tempting. However, without any carbohydrate additives, again, intake is likely to be self-limited. So, for breakfast, it is better to go for fruits such as blueberries and a boiled egg rather than cereals.

Most authors of diet books emphasize that it is important not to skip meals. Remember, the overall strategy is to reduce calorie intake. It is important not to exchange the omission of breakfast for eating late at night, which is really bad news.

Create a curfew at 8 PM, and don't eat after that, except on special occasions. Drink water at any time in large volumes; the more, the better. Avoid too much caffeine, which stimulates the appetite. However, drink as much calorie-free liquid as possible. Tea and coffee are okay in moderation. But, if you need a sweetener, use sugar-free ones such as Splenda.

Lunch and dinner are necessary! Go for grilled foods and throw away the frying pan. If you don't have one, you can't use it, and this will help. Look at the labels on meats in the supermarket and go for those with high protein and low fat, such as turkey or chicken breast and white meat.

Pork is acceptable, but cut off the surrounding fat. Fish is excellent, again, grilled without batter or breadcrumbs. But it has unfortunately become increasingly expensive.

Green-and-white is the color scheme of choice. So, add to the white meat or fish, green vegetables such as broccoli, asparagus, green beans, lettuce, and Brussels sprouts. Add olive oil to moisten it.

For white vegetables, onions are great; you can eat as many as you like. However, potatoes are bad, French fries in particular. Bread is also out; just don't eat it. Triscuits, particularly the low-fat ones, are acceptable, and Ryvita is good.

Add some butter to these and a small amount of jelly or jam if you are hungry, such as blueberry jam. It is excellent! Raspberry or blackcurrant is also acceptable, but not great. Grapes are just sugar. The other red or black fruits are nutritionally valuable.

Avoid desserts while you are trying to lose weight. Alcohol in moderation is acceptable. Red wine is best. Alcohol should be restricted to two drinks a day, though it is probable that a small amount is beneficial.

A combined multivitamin and mineral preparation should be taken daily. The large pharmacy chains probably produce the least expensive of these, which gives comprehensive nutritional coverage.

Exercise is a very important adjunct to dieting. Walk whenever it is feasible to do so, and try to walk three miles per day. Cycling is an excellent form of exercise, burning up to 350 to 400 calories per hour. It is feasible to walk and cycle for relatively long periods of time without damaging joints. This form of exercise is also less boring, and the scenery can frequently be changed.

Joining a gym is excellent, and working out with weights is beneficial; it stimulates the body to produce muscle rather than fat. And this, in turn, improves overall fitness, exercise tolerance, and mental as well as physical well-being. In general, make every effort to stay active;

getting out into the company and mixing with friends is good. Sitting on the couch in front of the television watching fast food advertisements is bad. In fact, it is the root cause of so much of the present-day obesity explosion.

Medication can be helpful for those who are struggling to achieve success with diet alone. As indicated, radical advances have recently been made in the efficacy of the drugs used to reduce weight. And these drugs may also be beneficial in terms of reducing heart attacks and strokes.

For those who are 100 pounds or more overweight, surgery is an option. Although there are risks associated with surgery, the risk of continuing in the obese state is greater than those associated with the operative procedure. Therefore, these risks are currently worth taking.

But with the advent of the new powerful drugs such as Wegovy, the amount of surgery required may be significantly reduced. The major question underlying the management of obesity at the moment will rest on the short and long-term success of the new drugs being introduced.

CONCLUSION

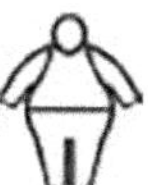

The development of the new class of drugs, the semaglutides, has produced astounding results with weight losses comparable to those achieved by weight-reducing surgery. It has undoubtedly had a significant impact on the successful treatment of Type 2 diabetes.

Overall, they must be anticipated as being safer and potentially more convenient and compliant than the major high-risk surgical procedures. These procedures are typically performed for the morbidly obese patient. Should a regain in weight occur, as is very common following surgical procedures, further therapy with these drugs can be given. This will naturally result in further weight loss. These drugs stand on the threshold of challenging and possibly replacing a large amount of high-risk bariatric surgery!

ABOUT THE AUTHOR

Dr. Tom Taylor is a retired surgeon who was a consultant surgeon at Manchester Royal infirmary and later Professor of surgery in the Michael E De Bakey Department of Surgery at Baylor College of Medicine in Houston, Texas. Throughout his many years of surgical practice he gained broad experience in the management of problems and complications related to surgical conditions where the fundamental underlying problem related to bad diet and obesity.

He believes that it is vital to fight the 12 major killers that are the threats to longevity in the present day society, 11 of which are fundamentally related to eating a bad diet and being overweight, obese or diabetic. In this text he emphasizes an understanding of the causes of these conditions and the way in which their prevalence can be reduced and deferred, thereby improving lifestyle and increasing longevity.

Taylor has written 12 books including, Upper Digestive Surgery, Surgical Gastroenterology, Case Studies in General Surgery, Pelvic Pouch Procedures, Overcoming Obesity, Lifestyle and Longevity and Honoring Holistic Health Habits. He has written over 100 scientific papers and held 10 US patents.

He lives in Cheshire, England and Houston Texas. His interests are singing, cricket, football and railways.

www.ingramcontent.com/pod-product-compliance
Lightning Source LLC
Chambersburg PA
CBHW052113030426
42335CB00025B/2968

* 9 7 8 1 9 7 0 7 1 1 3 1 8 *